OUTLIER

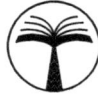

PALMETTO
PUBLISHING
Charleston, SC
www.PalmettoPublishing.com

Paperback ISBN: 9798822963221
eBook ISBN: 9798822963238

OUTLIER

One couple's story of life and love and Glioblastoma

TIM ANGELL

For Debbie Lee

Prologue

The following story is written with as much attention to timeline as possible, though since it covers fifty years of our lives, I have had to wrap some details around each other to save from boring the reader.

I first met Debbie Kessler when she was in seventh grade and I was in eighth grade. I had just moved to Moscow, PA. My father had changed jobs and was teaching psychology at the University of Scranton. One of my newfound friends was Rob Walsh, and we were standing in the front foyer of North Pocono High School one morning with another new friend, Dave Gardener.

As we waited for the school bell to tell us we could move to our locker and classes, a friend of Rob's named Tom came by and Rob introduced me to him and his girlfriend, Debbie Kessler. To this day, Debbie and I remember this moment and often relate it to people about how we met.

Four years later, after seeing Debbie now and then around school and at school activities, but not hanging out together, Debbie and I shared a mixed class study hall. She ended up sitting right in front of me, and we got to know each other a little better. At one point, she told me she had broken up with her boyfriend Tom over a disagreement about what Debbie needed to do for Tom. Debbie was sixteen and I was seventeen when we shared that study hall. I could see she was strong-willed even then. I liked that.

We met after school on the sidewalk in front of the gymnasium. She talked about her old boyfriend and her family. I listened. Being a psychologist's son, I knew listening was a good thing to do to get someone to open up to you.

Debbie was pretty and very opinionated. I was surprised she event spoke to me. She was also very talented. She made her own clothes, she was crafty, and she was smart. When I finally got the nerve to ask her out, Debbie told me she would have to ask her mother. Later, she told me this was not really true, but she was not sure if she wanted to go out with me. I was a nerd. I was in the band at school, playing trombone and bassoon. I was a skinny kid, too, weighing about a hundred-twenty pounds.

But I was determined to go out with Debbie, and she did not actually say, "No," so I kept asking. She finally said yes. Debbie was my first date. I was so excited to tell my mother that I had a date. She knew already that I liked Debbie and that we had been talking.

Our first date was on Friday, September 21, 1973, and it was great! We went to see the movie *Godspell*, a musical interpretation of the gospel. It was very uplifting and the music was great. We went to Papa's Pizza in downtown Scranton after the movie. When I took her home and was ready to go, she kissed me. She often laughed when telling this story to friends over the years that I was shaking as we kissed. I always say it was because it was a little chilly.

I worked at Stephen's Drug Store in Moscow all through high school. So, I had a little money to go out with. Debbie worked at the Tasty Freeze ice cream shop in Daleville, just up the road from Moscow. Working around our busy school, work, and activity schedules, we went on a few more dates. We liked each other, though she thought I was weird. I thought she was a wild one.

One time, shortly after we started dating, Debbie called me in a panic. "Come and get me. I'm not at home. I jumped out my bedroom window and I am at a neighbor's. It's a long story."

Of course, I went and got her. Saved her. I was a knight in shining armor that night. It turned out that she had been arguing with her sisters at home, and everyone was angry, so she had locked herself in her room and climbed out the window. She ran to the neighbors' house and called me. She called me! I think I was hooked from then on.

Debbie came from a large family. She had two older sisters, Tina and Terri, twins. She had a sister a year younger, Sandy. Then, there was Lesa, four years younger, and little Eddie, who was only four years old when we started dating. Her father's mother also lived with the family, Grandma Kessler.

Debbie had hundreds of cousins, aunts, and uncles, all of whom lived around the area. It seemed like everyone

I knew at school turned out to be related to her in some way. This was far different from my own family, made up of me, my brother Phil, three years younger, and my sister Heather, seven years younger. We had no other family in the area and not too many elsewhere.

Our families and upbringing were so very different. Debbie and I were different in many ways, but somehow very complimentary, even in the beginning. She was outgoing and flirty. I was nerdy and reserved. She was crafty and I was intellectual. As we spent more time together, we brought out many sides of each other. Our union was greater than either of us individually.

Soon, we were inseparable. We dated exclusively right from the beginning. As the year went on, we spent more and more time together. I was a senior that year and Debbie a junior. We went to my prom. We talked on the phone for hours. We marched in parades and football games together. (Debbie was in the color guard during marching season.)

Through the next summer we spent as much time together as we could. We hiked and had picnics. We went to the movies and took rides. Debbie and I enjoyed each other's company in everything we did with each other.

In the fall, Debbie started her senior year of high school, and I started college at the University of Scranton. We continued dating. I even had the chance to play trombone at a few of the high school football games with the marching band. These were good times.

I did not care much for college. I passed through my semester without much studying and found most of the classes boring. I liked the literature and writing classes most, but they were not in my major, psychology, so they meant less for my future (so I thought then).

Debbie and I went to her semi-formal dance in December, dressed in matching outfits. She wore an orange dress with a brown vest handmade by her. I wore a brown blazer with an orange shirt. We felt well matched in every way.

Debbie had not been feeling too well lately and she went to the doctor. A letter sent from the doctor to her home, opened by her parents, told them all she was pregnant! That was not the way we thought things would go. Debbie called me and I went right over to the house. There was chaos in the house, so we went up to the front living room to sit together for a moment. I had bought Debbie a friendship ring with an aquamarine stone in it a few months previously. As we sat in the front room, I asked if she would remove that ring (which scared the crap out of her and I was sorry for it later). I then asked her if she would marry me, and I put the now engagement ring back on her finger. She said yes. She said yes.

We were married on January 10, 1975. I was never happier in my life than I was at that moment. I knew Debbie was the girl for me, and now we were together forever. We wore the same outfits we had worn to the semi-formal the month before.

Debbie was determined to finish high school and she did so with a flourish. She continued to do well in her classes and worked on the yearbook committee. She grew bigger as springtime blossomed. There were challenges with some of the teachers who thought she should not be there. But Debbie persevered. I remember one evening Debbie came home upset that a teacher who I had really respected had ridiculed her in class and said she should not be there. I called the teacher at home and told him that we were doing together what we thought was right and Debbie should be respected for that. I said I had always respected him and hoped that he would do the same for us. That ended the problems with teachers, and Debbie never had another issue with anyone that I know about.

Debbie graduated from North Pocono in June. She gave birth to our first son, Aaron, on July 1st. We were parents. Debbie was eighteen and I was nineteen. I believe we were both ready, though it did feel a little precarious at times. We had each other, though, and it was us against the world.

Debbie and I moved seven times over the course of the next four years. We lived in two houses in Moscow; a camper at the Kessler homestead; two houses in Williamsport, PA; a house in West Hartford, CT; and finally, a house in Winsted, CT. We moved from job to job, both of us working to keep things together. Unbeknownst to us, Debbe was pregnant as we moved to Connecticut from Williamsport.

Once we moved to Winsted, things became more stable. I had a job at Ovation instruments, maker of the famous round-back guitar. Debbie was working as the manager of a small boutique clothing store on Union Place in Hartford. She had gotten this job through my mother, who was friends with the store owner. Debbie's knowledge of clothing and sewing was helpful in her work there. Aaron accompanied her to the store every day, since he was still too young for school.

For months, Debbie continued to commute to Hartford daily to work in the boutique. As her pregnancy progressed, this became more difficult. The summer heat in the city was brutal and the twenty-five-mile drive in traffic was challenging. She kept it up as long as she could until near the due date and then gave her notice.

Brian, our youngest son, was born in November of 1979, just eight months after our move from Williamsport. We lived in a rental duplex with the owners upstairs and us downstairs. The Brochu family was very nice and we stayed there six years. They treated us much like family. At one point, they asked if their son could move into our apartment and we began a quick search for a house we could afford.

In 1985, Debbie and I bought our house, the same one we live in now. The boys were little, still. Aaron was ten and Brian was six. When we bought the house, everything needed to be done to it. It was a two-family home. We took over the upstairs apartment right away, and in three weeks we painted all the walls and cleaned up everything to make it livable. Then, when the downstairs tenant moved out after not paying rent for six months, we took that over and renovated it. Four months later, we moved downstairs and began renting out the upstairs.

After Brian's birth, Debbie took some waitress jobs in local restaurants. This worked for a while, but neither of us liked the lifestyle of me working days and Debbie working nights. Once Brian was old enough to be taken care of in day-care, Debbie went looking for daytime work. She found a job at the Hitchcock Chair company in Riverton. The first job there was chair assembly, which she found she was very good at. She soon learned table and cabinet assembly and later on finishing.

Later, after owning our house for about five years, we asked the tenants about finding another place so we could take over the whole house. The boys needed more room. Our tenants were great and told us they were actually buying a house soon and were planning to tell us shortly, so it worked out perfectly.

Debbie ran for schoolboard that fall and won the election. She served for four years on the board, learning a great deal about politics and the school district. She was an excellent and thorough board member and worked very hard on the budgets and human resources issues. She stepped down after four years in order to work on other things. She remained a very active member of the Republican Party for all of her years after this experience, eventually becoming Treasurer and Chair of the local chapter. Later on, she became a moderator for elections and continued to work closely with elected officials. That never stopped.

About this time, Debbie was struck by the idea of becoming an Emergency Medical Technician. Hitchcock Chair was looking for a few employees to take the course and become EMTs for their company. They could also volunteer to work with the New Hartford Ambulance if they desired. Debbie thought this would be a rewarding and positive thing to be involved with, and so she took the training. She helped with many incidents at work and took on many night and weekend shifts at the ambulance headquarters. She found it to be very exciting, and she helped many people during the time that Hitchcock was in business.

Just after Christmas, in 1986, Debbie's dad passed away suddenly. This was a shock to the entire family. Debbie was just twenty-nine years old and it affected her deeply. It also cemented the desire to help people as and EMT. She always felt that she might have been able to do something for her dad if she was there at the time he suffered his heart attack, and she vowed to be there for whoever she could be after that.

As the boys grew and became more active, we enrolled them in Cub Scouts and then Boy Scouts. This was a great time for our family. Debbie convinced me to get involved, too, first at the committee level and soon as an assistant

Scout Master. I enjoyed being with the boys at campouts and meetings. It gave us time to be together doing activities both they and I enjoyed.

I took on the role of Scoutmaster and held that for four years. In our troop, we scheduled a campout for every month of the year. Some of the most adventurous times were when we camped in the middle of winter. The boys built snow shelters and camped in them. We came home after those campouts with tall tales of how cold it got overnight and how we kept warm by a giant fire. The boys and I learned a lot about ourselves and about being prepared for anything. That mindset has proven to be very valuable over the many years since.

I was invited to join the local lodge of the Benevolent and Protective Order of Elks in 1985. A friend of the family from church recommended me, and with Debbie's blessing I joined the order. I became active right away, stepping into a low-level officer position later that Spring. I had never been very extroverted, so this experience was all new. I found that I liked being involved in the programs our local lodge put on, and it gave me a place to learn how to act in front of people. I found a new side of me that I did not know existed. I continued to advance through the various offices of the lodge and eventually became the lodge president, Exalted Ruler, in 1993. Debbie enjoyed attending lodge functions, too, and it became a second family to us. Debbie was able to join in 1996, after the national level determined that women could join.

As the 1990s flowed by, Debbie and I involved ourselves more with the Elks and Scouts. The boys were growing up. Aaron graduated from high school in 1993. He had high expectations of what to do with his life, too. Aaron entered the US Naval Academy in the summer of 1993, turning eighteen and joining the Navy on the same day, July 1, 1993.

As Aaron joined the Academy, Debbie and I joined the Naval Academy Parents Club of Connecticut. The Parent's Club was a great way for parents of midshipmen (the name given to Academy students), to be involved in Academy activities and keep in better touch with their children while they were at the school. We became active in the Parents Club as Aaron moved through the years at the Academy. Eventually, in 1997, Debbie and I were elected to co-presidents of our chapter in Connecticut.

1997, was a big year for the Angells. Aaron graduated from the Naval Academy and Brian from Gilbert High School in Winsted. The entire family, extending to grandparents and close friends, traveled to Annapolis, MD, to attend the week of festivities surrounding Aaron's graduation ceremony. It marked a high point in our lives to be involved at the level we all had reached. Aaron had chosen to enter the Marine Corps after graduation. He was chosen as the top Marine graduate that year and was presented with a special award at one of the many ceremonies that happened during graduation week. We were so proud when he stepped up to the stage to receive a specially made sword from the family of retired General Buce.

Brian's graduation at Gilbert School was also well-attended by family and friends. He chose a different path than Aaron, as always. Brian attended Bridgewater State University in Massachusetts, where he majored in flight. He wanted to be a pilot, and that was one of the few state schools in the country that had flight as a major. He began pilot training the first year he entered in the fall of 1997.

While at the Naval Academy, Aaron met another midshipman who would change his life. Megan Mastell was a first-year midshipman (known at that time as a plebe) when Aaron was moving from sophomore to junior. Megan was attached to a detail that Aaron was responsible for training during the summer. There are many stories they can talk about the next two years of working together, though they were not a couple during the time Aaron was in the school.

After Aaron graduated, he kept in close contact with Megan, and they began seeing each other socially. Aaron invited Megan to accompany him to the annual Marine Corps birthday ball. They soon found that they were happy together and the relationship grew ever stronger. During Megan's senior year at the Academy, Aaron asked her to marry him. Their wedding was held in the Academy chapel, just two days after Megan graduated. Both the Mastell family and the Angell family were thrilled to be involved in the ceremony and celebration.

Aaron and Megan have moved around the country ever since that day, while building a family of their own. Megan served our country in the Navy for five years, concentrating on weather forecasting in the Norfolk Atlantic Weather Service, tracking hurricanes and storms throughout the Atlantic Ocean and reporting to Navy ships at sea. Aaron advanced through many ranks and positions in the Marine Corps and is currently a Colonel.

Brian met a girl at Bridgewater who changed his life. Liz was a student in the special education program at the university. They quickly became an item, and Brian's focus changed from flying to things on the ground and closer to home. He ultimately graduated from Bridgewater with a major in business administration and an art minor. Soon after graduating, Brian began working as a teacher in a special education private school.

Brian found that he loved teaching and went on to finish a master's degree in education and went to work in the Boston area as a middle school teacher. Liz also finished her master's degree and worked in the special education area in Boston.

Brian and Liz were married in Dorchester, MA, in August of 2002 and bought a home there that same year. They still live in the same house and have raised their three beautiful children there.

Debbie had worked for many years at the Hitchcock Chair company. She had advanced through many positions there. She was a group leader in the assembly department. She learned stenciling from the old masters who had worked there for many years. Debbie's talent for crafts enabled her to catch onto the stenciling quickly, and she filled in when people were not there or when extra help was needed.

Debbie eventually learned so much about all the aspects of furniture-making that she became a traveling repair person for Hitchcock. She had her own van with tools and finishing supplies and would roll up to customers' homes and fix scratches, dents, cracks, and gaps in their furniture without the need to take the items back to the factory. She loved this job most of any of the work she did for Hitchcock. It gave her a chance to use all her talents and skills. She continued this position until the Hitchcock company closed its doors in 2006, after a long struggle to compete with foreign competition in the furniture business.

In 1999, I moved from the Ovation factory in New Hartford to the headquarters of Kaman Music Corporation in Bloomfield. I had an opportunity to use the skills I had gained in computer management, such as database programming and spreadsheets.

The next couple of years were a time when Debbie and I got used to living on our own as a couple, the first time since we were married. We did a lot with the local Elks Lodge and with the State Elks. I took on the position of vice president of the State Elks and then president in 2004. Debbie was by my side throughout that great adventure.

My work at Kaman Music continued through 2010. However, Hitchcock did not fare well in the 2000s and was out of business in 2006. This opened the door for Debbie's next challenge. When Hitchcock closed, there was an opportunity for Debbie to attend college and get her two-year degree as part of a state program for displaced employees.

At the same time Hitchcock closed, Debbie decided to move her EMT work to the Winsted Area Ambulance Association. She took on many shifts and made hundreds of calls over the next several years. She loved the work and helping others. Later on, she ran for treasurer position and held that post for many years as well.

Debbie took great advantage of the government retraining program and was able to attend and ultimately graduate with an associate's degree in business management from the local community college. She graduated in 2008 with honors.

After graduation, Debbie went to work for a moving company in Torrington as their office manager. She enjoyed the work for a time but found that working there was causing her stress. The owners were not of the same mind as Debbie in terms of how things should be done, and she felt uncomfortable with the processes.

So, Debbie moved on. To tide things over and have time to do some of the family things she wanted to be doing, Debbie got a job at Regional Refuse Disposal District 1 in New Hartford. She was the gatekeeper who checked people in, just part-time at first. She loved it! She was stationed in a little building at the entrance and was able to welcome people into the facility, check their annual stickers, and sell stickers to those who did not have them. This suited her nicely. She stayed in that position for about two years. Debbie often looked back on those days with fond memories, recounting the times she sat in that building as the snow fell outside and the wood fire warmed her up.

In 2014, the RRDD1 administrator decided to retire. Jim was his name, and he came to Debbie with an application for that position and told her she should apply. She was very reluctant to give up the job she was doing. She did not want to be the administrator. Jim convinced her to put in for the job.

During the interview, Debbie told the Board of Directors that she was not sure she wanted to take on the responsibilities of this position. They asked what it would take for her to do it. Debbie told them she would work four days a week, not Saturday. She wanted to be able to have weekends to visit the grandkids. The Board accepted her requirements and chose her as the new administrator.

Debbie took the position in 2014 and thrived in her new role. The employees liked her motherly methods. The Board liked her detail-oriented management techniques. She managed the budget, the federal programs, the equipment purchases; virtually everything at the facility was under her watchful eye. She grew to love it all.

While this was going on with Debbie in 2014, I was also going through major changes in my employment.

Kaman Music had sold to Fender Guitars in 2010 and was now being sold again. The new owners did not need the reporting support that I had been supplying to the company for the last fourteen years, so I was out of a job. Luckily, I landed back at another Kaman company. I took on a reporting management role at Kaman Industrial Technologies. It was a dream job for me. The money was better than ever, and I was working for a great manager who treated me with the utmost respect.

The next five years went on with Debbie and I growing closer and with our respective jobs being very fulfilling for us. We traveled a bit through these years, taking some cruises with family and seeing some other countries we did not expect to ever see. It was a loving time for us.

Perhaps our greatest trip ever was to Paris in 2018 over the Christmas holiday. We stayed in the Latin Quarter in a hotel that was built in 1380. We calculated that we walked over forty miles that week throughout the city. We saw everything we hoped for and more. The people we met were wonderful. I think this was the most special trip Debbie and I ever took together.

The following year, 2019, was a time of change. Debbie's mom was ill quite a bit of the year, in and out of the hospital and treatment facilities. Debbie traveled between Winsted and her mom's home in Springbrook every couple of weeks. She would leave our house after work on Tuesday and come back on Thursday night in order to be at work on Friday. She cherished the time with her mom and wanted to help in any way she could.

Henrietta took a turn for the worse in November that year. Debbie spent as much time as she could with her. Finally, her mom entered the hospital with another infection near Thanksgiving. We headed there to be with the family in the hospital.

Once her mom's condition was somewhat stable, Debbie and I headed for New York City to be with Brian and Liz who had planned a Thanksgiving trip to see the Macy's Parade. It was a big deal as we were able to see it from the New York Athletic Club where the NYC Police Department had food and beverages and a special viewing section. Liz had a good friend who was high up in the department and had invited us all to participate. It was spectacular.

While we were there, we received a call from the hospital that things had made a turn for the worse. We left the city early and got back to the hospital on Sunday morning. The family was gathered and taking turns sitting with Henrietta. We took over the waiting room and lounged out there when we were not in the hospital room with her. This was just before COVID, and there were not the rules for gathering or visiting that we all are familiar with today.

After another rally from her mom, Debbie and I determined we could do nothing more at the hospital, and we reluctantly headed home to Winsted on Sunday night. We both worked on Monday and then settled in for the night.

Late that night, Henrietta passed away and her struggles were over. She had fought a battle with numerous medical issues over several years, and her body finally had enough.

We headed back to Springbrook for the funeral, as did all of the children and grandchildren of Henrietta. The funeral was held on a sunny day in December, and many beautiful sentiments were shared by family and friends. The only child who was missing was Terri, twin sister of Tina, who was not able to come from Florida due to her own failing health.

Debbie was quite depressed after the passing of her mother. The Christmas season was not quite as sweet as it always was for her that year. The new year brought with it the first news about a new virus that was popping up here and there, often killing the individuals or small groups of people who caught it. COVID was the name given, and it struck fear in everyone.

By March, the whole world was beginning to fear this illness. What was it? How did it pass from one person to the next? Who would it strike next? We lived in fear. We began to shut ourselves in, trying to avoid catching the sickness as hospitals filled up and the news of the day counted the dead.

News from Florida about Debbie's sister Terri was not good. She was in and out of the hospital. Sisters Sandy and Lesa went down to visit and try to help as they could. Over the weekend of March 28th and 29th, Terri took a turn for the worse. She had recently been diagnosed with lung cancer on top of the other breathing issues she was plagued with. It was determined that she would need to be on a ventilator to keep her going, and the family gathered around her to see what she would do. Terri decided that she no longer wanted to fight. Terri decided to be disconnected from the machines. She spent her last day with family around, writing notes to them since she was unable to speak. Her spirits seemed good and her mood was steady. As the sun went down outside the hospital, the machines were turned off. Terri had said her goodbyes to her sisters and children. She passed quietly within just a few minutes. It was March 30th, Debbie's birthday.

Debbie was devastated by her sister's passing. The fact it was on her birthday made it even more distressing. We could do nothing from Winsted. Nobody could travel due to COVID. There could not even be a proper funeral for family and friends to attend. The hospital arranged for a time for the family to say their last goodbyes in a visiting room, though nobody could come close to Terri. Her children shared what they could via FaceTime, and everyone wept at the sadness of the situation.

During the next several months, Debbie worked fiercely to keep her employees safe at RRDD1. They had to remain open during the time when most businesses shut down due to COVID. Debbie searched around to find protective equipment the employees could use to keep from passing the virus. She developed methods to keep employees at safe distances from each other and customers.

RRDD1 remained open throughout the year without any COVID infections. This was no doubt due to the diligence Debbie exhibited during that time.

Debbie also continued working with the ambulance as an attendant on ambulance calls and as the assistant to the treasurer. She never wavered from that duty to her crew and the ambulance association. We and two other good friends at the Elks Lodge even sewed over ninety Tyvek aprons for use by ambulance attendants when it was found that aprons were not available.

As the spring and summer rolled on, it became very challenging for Debbie to find the equipment needed to protect her employees. She spent countless hours searching the internet for suppliers. She complained of headaches during this time and was sure they were caused by the stress she was experiencing. Somehow, she found the items she needed.

We spent as much time as we could at home where we were safe. We only went out to work or to help at the Elks Lodge that had come up with an idea to sell dinners curbside to members. Members would drive up to the front of the lodge, and we would hand them their pre-ordered dinners and collect the money with no contact.

I was soon told that my reporting team should work from home, and I did that as another safeguard to not spread the virus. This, I continued until my retirement.

As summer waned its way into September, some family activities were beginning to take place again. We carefully chose which ones we would participate in. One event was coming up that we had to attend. Our grandchildren Abigail and Joseph were to take their first holy communion in September and we decided to go. This would be in late September.

Table of Contents

CHAPTER 1

September 28, 2020 – The Beginning

Saturday morning, September 28, 2020, was a beautiful morning in Boston. Debbie and I were visiting our son Brian and his wife Liz for the weekend to celebrate the first holy communion of our two youngest grandchildren, Joseph and Abigail. Their older brother Patrick was excited for the day as well.

The Catholic church was glowing as the sun shone through its colorful stained-glass windows, and the ceremony was sweet. The family headed out to the side lawn for photos, and smiles were broad as the twins stood tall in their finest church outfits.

We all headed back to the house, Patrick in our little red convertible, talking away in the back seat as Grandma talked about the upcoming party. We pulled into our parking spot in front of the house. Debbie said something quite strange and unintelligible as she stepped out of the car and held the seat back forward so Patrick could climb out.

I asked Debbie, "What was that? What did you say?"

She answered, "Oh, I don't know. I'm too hot."

We crossed the street toward the house and she faltered a bit. I grabbed her for a second to steady her.

Debbie said, "I think I just need to go downstairs for a minute. I'm not feeling too well. Please don't say anything." And we headed into the house and down to the basement where our room was. I went with her, feeling a little concerned. Debbie went straight into the bathroom, but emerged only a few moments later looking a bit dazed.

"Are you alright?" I asked.

I noticed she was wavering, and she said something under her breath and it was not really words that I could pick out. The right side of her face was drooping and she licked her lips as she stood holding onto a rocking chair. I pulled her forward and sat her down, looking into her eyes. They were glassy and staring a bit, not really focusing on anything in particular.

I ran to the top of the stairs and out to the yard where the party for the twins was just getting started.

"Brian," I yelled. "Call 911. I think Mom might be having a stroke!" We were running back down as he pressed the emergency number on his cell phone. I found Debbie sitting where I left her. She was murmuring something that we could not understand. More alarmed by the second, I sat with her, and we waited the few minutes it took for an ambulance crew to arrive at the house.

Two emergency medical technicians came down the stairs with some of their equipment. They were young women, so it comforted me a bit. They came to Debbie and began their survey. She was still not speaking clearly. The EMT took her vitals, and the two immediately determined that we would need to use a special piece of equipment that Debbie could sit in and be lifted up the stairs. Nobody wanted her to attempt to walk up the stairs.

The stairs were quite tight, and we ended up having to have Brian stand above the EMT up the stairs from Debbie while I stood below the other EMT. The four of us lifted her up the tight stairs with quite some difficulty, and at one point we were stopped. Debbie, who was an EMT with our local volunteer ambulance service for nearly twenty years, was now attempting to manage the situation and tell these two Boston EMTs that she needed to stand up and get to the top of the steps herself. After some discussion and a bit more maneuvering, we managed to get her into the kitchen at the top of the stairs and then quickly outside to a waiting stretcher.

As Debbie was moved onto the stretcher, I noticed a certain stare, some call it the one-thousand-mile stare. Her eyes were glassy and not focused on anything in particular. She was not talking. The EMTs moved her around to the rear of the ambulance and pushed the stretcher in as the wheels collapsed underneath. This was the first year of COVID, and protocols in the healthcare field had been changed to protect everyone from too much close contact. I asked about riding with them but was told that was not possible and that I would be called by the hospital when it was determined what was happening and when I could come to be with Debbie.

The ambulance pulled away with lights and sirens. As they rounded the corner at the end of the street, we were all left breathless and attempting to process what had just happened. The grandchildren had been kept around the back of the house during the extrication, so we headed through the side yard into the party.

What the hell just happened?!

I was stunned. From my limited training for emergency medical situations, it appeared that Debbie had suffered a stroke. Her face had gone limp on the right side. Her right arm and leg were not working normally. She was not communicative. What happened?

This sudden attack was the beginning of this chapter in the story of Debbie Angell, an outlier.

About forty-five minutes later, I received a cell phone call from Debbie's phone. It was the emergency room doctor at Boston University Medical Center, who had used the emergency button on Debbie's phone that called my phone. The doctor said that she was to be admitted. I asked if they had administered the special drug that had been developed to treat stroke victims during the first hour. He answered no that she had not suffered a stroke. It was some sort of seizure, and she had experienced another seizure in the emergency room. He said they were sending her for a CT scan and that if I wished to come to the hospital I could. Only I could come at this time because COVID protocol was in full effect. The hospital was experiencing a major upsurge in COVID cases. He told me to come in through the ER entrance, and they would clear me to come to wherever she would be at the time.

Brian drove me to the hospital and dropped me off. He headed back home since it would likely be hours before I would return.

It took some time to get through the COVID screening and to find out where Debbie was. By this time, she had been moved up to the Neuro ICU department. I was allowed to go to the waiting room outside that department and wait for further news and instruction. When I got to that room, I was the only person there. It was about 3:00 p.m.

As I waited, I moved around the room, unable to sit still. Worry had set in by this time and my mind was racing. In one of the chairs, I found a quarter, nickel, and two pennies. Change. I had a silly thought for a moment that I don't need change, not right now. Odd thoughts in such a time and place.

Finally, a nurse came in and said Debbie was settled and I could come into her room to see her. I followed the nurse through the halls and to a room with an outside viewing area for the nurse on duty. As I looked through that window, I could see machines and Debbie's small form tucked into a hospital bed. We entered the room. Debbie had been intubated! This quite shocked me. No one had told me of this. For a moment, I thought about Debbie's previous discussions about not being kept alive on machines. I bit my tongue as I knew an explanation would come.

The nurse explained that the emergency department had intubated Debbie to ensure a clear airway. They were worried that the seizures could close that down and she would not be able to breathe. She assured me that this was just a precaution and that once Debbie was stabilized, they would be able to remove the tubes, probably within twenty-four hours. It was still a shock, though.

Dr. C., the head of neurology, came in next. He said that Debbie had experienced another seizure in the ED while the team was working with her. He explained that they had given her Keppra, a drug to stop seizures, but that she had an allergic reaction to it. She had a rash and reddened face. I presume this was what prompted the intubation.

Dr. C. went on to say that the initial scan showed what the ED team believed might be a brain bleed. However, he told me he had a different interpretation. He flipped on the computer screen and opened a program with the scan view on it. He pointed out an area in the right front of Debbie's brain that he believed was a mass, not a bleed. He was careful not to read too much into that initial scan and said that as soon as they could extubate Debbie, they planned to have a more comprehensive MRI done. This would likely be Sunday night. For now, this was all the information he could give me, and he said that I could certainly stay in the room for the remainder of visiting hours. Unfortunately, due to COVID, I could not stay overnight, though.

Dr. C. said that he would be checking in throughout the night and he would leave me with her for now. The nurse stayed with me and we talked a bit. She told me that they had taken off Debbie's jewelry and glasses and put them in her purse, which had been taken to the security locker in the administration office for safe keeping. She said they had tried to remove Debbie's rings but had not been able to do it because they were too tight. She called in another nurse who was actually a specialist in this sort of thing and had some tricks for removing rings without cutting them off. Vaseline and dental floss did the trick, and I was able to take Debbie's rings with me.

I sat in the darkened room for a while, listening to the machinery click and pump oxygen. Debbie did not stir. The moment was almost too much to manage, and my mind continued to race. So, Debbie had not had a stroke. She had seizures probably caused by that mass in her brain.

Later in the coming days, Debbie told me that she had known she was having a seizure in the basement of Brian's house and had told us that was what had happened. That was the murmuring she was making that we could not understand. Her years of working as a volunteer EMT had told her that. I thought it amazing that she could have remembered anything from those first moments of the incident.

Finally, at about 8:00 p.m. it was time for me to go. That was very difficult. I felt exhausted and frightened for my sweet girl. Brian was waiting for me and so I kissed Debbie on the cheek. I told her I would be back as soon as they would let me in the next day and that she would be OK.

As I climbed into Brian's vehicle outside the hospital, I'm sure he could see the worry on my face. Brian was a great comfort as we headed for his house just a few minutes away from the hospital. When we arrived at the house, Liz was waiting for us, and we sat and talked about what had happened in the hospital. I had a drink to settle my nerves and we sat for a while. I was worried about how the kids had reacted to the experience and they told me they were OK. All they knew at this time was that Grandma got sick and had to go to the hospital. It had been a day that none of us would ever forget. Change was in the air. I headed down to the basement bedroom and crawled into bed. I laid awake for a long time that night.

CHAPTER 2

Sunday, September 27th - Day Two

COVID protocol at that time in a big city hospital was very tight indeed. All visitors had to go through a checkpoint to be questioned about symptoms before even being admitted into the main waiting area. Visiting hours had been curtailed too. Just one person could visit per day. The times were just from 2:00 p.m. to 8:00 p.m., no exceptions. Long lines were the norm and patience was required. The faces of other visitors showed the strain. Once you reached the visitors desk after the COVID check, the attendant would take your name and give you a nametag. Only then were you allowed to proceed to the floor of your loved one and wait in that waiting room for access to the patient's room. This whole process took nearly an hour every day.

That second day as I entered Debbie's room, I saw the tubes piled up on the floor in the corner and Debbie was awake. She was very happy to see me. I gave her a kiss and pulled up a chair to be near the bed. She was still medicated and was having some difficulty realizing where she was and what was happening. We talked a little about what she knew of the time since she had been picked up in the ambulance. She critiqued the ambulance attendant's actions and complained about the stair chair not being used properly. I took this as a good sign. She had not lost her critical thinking abilities.

The doctor came in again and we discussed what we knew and what would be happening. An MRI was scheduled for later that evening. Debbie had questions about the mass, but the doctor could not elaborate much further without the MRI. So, we sat and talked for the next several hours. Debbie slept some of the time as the stress of the situation got to her. I looked out the window at the street below.

When visiting hours were ending, it was hard to leave. Debbie wanted me to stay, but that would not be possible. Separation in these difficult times was very hard on both of us. I assured her that I would be back as soon as they would let me in. Unfortunately, Debbie's purse was still locked up so we could not leave her phone with her, so the nurse assured me she would call if there were any issues or if Debbie needed to tell me something.

CHAPTER 3

Monday, September 28th – Testing and Prep

Liz had put together a care package for me to take into Debbie. There was a pink journal for her to write in. There were pictures from the kids. There was her favorite bathrobe that we had gotten from the Bellagio Hotel in Las Vegas, and a cute set of gators for her to wear when she got up. The pictures went up on the wall immediately, and Debbie's eyes sparkled a bit to see the work from the kids.

The MRI had been done overnight and more information was now available. The mass was a tumor of some sort, though we did not yet know what type. More testing would need to be done. Debbie was on seizure medication, so it was believed that would help for the time being.

Over the next nine days, the doctors and technicians at BMC put Debbie through a number of tests to determine what was happening to her and what should be done.

There was an EEG to determine if she was experiencing any more seizures. There were no more seizures. This was considered a positive result of the medication being used to prevent those seizures.

There was a WADA test to determine how much of her communications and processing was being done on the left side of her brain. This particular test was done because she was a lefty and there was concern that her right side may actually be where most of the speaking and reading processes were taking place. It turned out that most of the usual left side processing was happening on the left side. This was important in the discussion of how aggressive the surgeon could be in removing tumor on the right side. Had the fact she was left-handed actually meant that the communication processing was on the right side of the brain, they would have had to be much more careful about touching anything to do with that.

Another MRI was to be done within forty-eight hours of surgery to map out the part of the brain in which the tumor was located. This would help the surgeons know exactly where to remove whatever they could, hopefully without damage to any surrounding tissue or functions.

I now know a bit of what Debbie was thinking during this period, as I read through her journal. She was afraid of being incapacitated as a result of the surgery. She mentioned several times that she did not want to be a burden to me or the family. She questioned why this was happening to her.

Debbie was sixty-three years old, though not many people would believe it. She had been a volunteer Emergency Medical Technician for over thirty years. She was the administrator of the local transfer station (dump) that served three towns in Northwest Connecticut. She was a co-owner of a pottery studio on Main Street in our town of Winsted. She was a proud grandmother of six grandchildren who she loved to entertain with craft projects and stories. She was the author of a book on recycling. All in all, she ran circles around most of the people around her, including me. Most of all she was a very loving person.

Debbie's personality was important for the challenges she was about to face. She was very positive and caring. She gave of her time and energy to any cause she believed in. She never let anything stop her from doing what she thought was right. We often laughed as a family because her pet name from her father growing up was "Goddamn Bullhead." She was strong-willed. That is for sure.

Back to the present. As the testing progressed and a clearer picture of what was happening began to develop, the doctors determined that the tumor must be removed as quickly as possible. They said to us that their objective was to remove all that they could, and Debbie should walk out of the hospital after a short recovery and be able to continue doing what she had been able to do before. We were scared but hopeful. Debbie's main surgeon, who Debbie always called Dr. D. because she could not pronounce his last name, made us feel confident that her surgery and recovery would go well.

CHAPTER 4

October 8, 2020 – Surgery

The day of neurosurgery was extremely stressful and long. I was not able to come to the hospital before the normal time, even though surgery was scheduled for around 11:00 a.m. This concerned me and was dreadful for Debbie, who by this time wanted me around her all of the time. However, when I got to the hospital, I found out that everything had been pushed back, and the staff was waiting to get everything lined up as it was needed. Surgery finally began at around 4:00, so I was able to be with Debbie for a while prior to them taking her to the operating suite. Debbie was calm and seemed confident that she would be fine after the operation.

Brain surgery is a slow and precise process, as everyone knows. After Debbie was taken out of her room, I was told we would be moving to the Neurological ICU after the surgery, and I could move all of Debbie's flowers and personal items up to that area so they would be there when she woke up. That gave me something to do and helped me get my mind off what was happening to her each moment. After moving her things, I was allowed to wait in the good old waiting room where I was that first night. I spent some time there and then took a walk to get something to eat. I also wanted to see if I could find the chapel.

As I wandered through a few hallways, probably looking a little bit dazed, a doctor asked if I was OK and if she could help with anything. I told her what was going on and that I was looking for the chapel. She directed me to it and bid me well.

As I entered the chapel, there was just one other person there, but it was uncomfortable because they were from a different religion than I am used to, and they had on their phone a video that seemed to be rather loud and aggressive, when all I wanted was peace and tranquility. After a little while, that person left me to my own thoughts, and it was very still in the chapel. I prayed that Debbie's doctors would have great skill and knowledge to take care of her and remove everything that was harming her. Once I finished my meditations, I left to get something to eat and returned to the waiting room.

That night, the visiting hours ending time came and went without anyone even suggesting that I should move from where I sat. Every once in a while, a nurse popped in to give me an update on the slow process that Debbie was undergoing. They were kind and caring, and it made me feel good that they wanted me to know it was going as expected.

Near 11:00 p.m. a nurse told me the operation had been completed and Debbie was being cleaned up and moved up to her room. I would be allowed to go in and see her for a few minutes before heading home. I exhaled and felt a great relief flow through my whole body. Once she was settled in the room, the nurse came and led me to her. There was a huge bandage wrapped around Debbie's head and she was sleeping. She slept peacefully, breathing silently and I held her hand. I left the hospital after midnight, and a security guard walked me to the parking garage. I was emotionally and physically exhausted from all that happened during that very long day.

CHAPTER 5

Recovery

The first day after surgery was spent in Neuro-ICU. Things were looking good for Debbie. Dr. D. reported that he removed about 98% of the tumor and was able to do it without disturbing much surrounding tissue. A biopsy would determine exactly what the tumor was, and we would know within a few days all that could be known. Debbie was in very good shape, due to her strong body and mental toughness. It was determined that she could be moved to a step-down unit the next day.

During the first couple of days after surgery, Debbie was very sensitive to light and sound, with sound especially bothersome. The step-down unit had so many bells and whistles around that Debbie complained of a lot of headaches. She became hyper-sensitive to her surroundings and could not get comfortable. So, within another day, she was moved out to the neuro-surgery floor, first to a room near the nurses' station, then to the end of the hall where the most peaceful rooms were located.

Headaches and a black eye on her right side were bothersome to her, and she found it difficult to settle down. Tylenol and some relaxing medication helped a bit and she slowly got through those first few days. After a couple of days of this, Debbie began to get back to normal, though a bit cranky, which I was happy about because it told me she was feeling better. Happily, her main concern became that I would bring her Dunkin Donuts coffee whenever I came to visit. This made us both smile.

Debbie was surrounded by love from her family and friends. She had seven flower arrangements all around her. We actually ran out of room on the windowsill at one point. She marveled that people had sent them to her and wrote in her journal that the flowers made her feel loved.

Debbie was able to change into her night gown and Bellagio robe, and that was of great comfort to her. She was even getting up to go to the bathroom and wash up now and then, though the nursing staff hated that and installed a motion detector in her bed to prevent her from getting up alone. I thought this was amusing, trying to control Debbie Angell in that way.

Five days out from surgery, another EEG test was performed and no ill effects were identified. She was having no seizures or other anomalous brain activity.

One week after surgery, the hospital tumor board met to discuss cases, including Debbie's. By this time the biopsy was completed and tumor pathology was known. Dr. D. and Dr. S., the neuro-oncologist assigned to Debbie, met with us in her room. They told us that the tumor had been identified as advanced glioblastoma multiform, methylated. Brain cancer. Shock went through our bodies.

Dr. S. took over the conversation and explained that there is a standard protocol to be followed, once Debbie was allowed to heal for four weeks. She would begin a chemo therapy and radiation treatment. This could be done back in Connecticut. Dr. S. recommended a neuro-oncologist at Yale in New Haven, and he would make contact with them if we wished.

After this meeting, we met again with neuro-surgeon Dr. D., who said that he recommended that Debbie be moved out, after a few more days, to a rehab facility in Connecticut via ambulance. Debbie balked at this, knowing so much about COVID issues in these facilities. She said that her best friend is a manager at the local Visiting Nurses in our town and that she wanted to go home. After some further discussion, this plan was approved and the Visiting Nurses of Litchfield were contacted to make arrangements.

On Friday, eight days after surgery, Debbie had had enough of BMC. She began by telling the nurse that she thought she should be checked out the next day. The nurse seemed encouraging about this and said she would speak with Dr. D. about it. Debbie reacted by stating that she wanted to be released the next day, for sure. I smiled knowing Debbie usually gets what she wants.

Early Saturday morning, well before I got to the hospital, Debbie called to tell me she would be getting out that day. The doctor on staff that day said he was not sure about this, and they would have to get Physical Therapy and Occupational Therapy approval prior to release. Debbie told them OK, but get it done.

I called my brother after Debbie's call and told him what was going on. Phil, my brother, told me to hold on and he would be up to pick me up and take us home to Connecticut. Too weak to refuse him, I said that would be fine. It actually was a lifesaver, as I do not know how I would have driven Debbie home alone. Phil picked me up within an hour and we headed in to the hospital. He brought with him a book to read in the car and said he would just wait for me to call on him to pick us up when we were ready.

By the time I got to the hospital for visiting hours, Debbie was sitting up in bed and complaining that nothing was happening. She was so ready to leave, after sitting there for twenty-one days. She pestered the doctor and nurses throughout the day, continuing to say she was leaving that day. I kept my brother apprised of the status throughout the day, apologizing for the delays. He said not to worry a bit; he was fine and prepared to wait.

Finally, Dr. D. was in the building and saw that things were not going so smoothly. It was after 4:00 p.m. and no movement had really taken place. PT and OT seemed on the fence about it, but finally it was determined that she could go. However, by this time, it was too late to get any of the medication Debbie would be needing the next morning from the hospital pharmacy. So, Dr. D. had the attending physician write the necessary prescriptions. Debbie was given just enough medications for that night.

By the time we finally got all of the approvals and paperwork done to get her out, it was 8:00 p.m. I called on Phil to bring the car around. We gathered up all of Debbie's remaining personal items and put her into a wheelchair for the escape to freedom. Dr. D. came in and wished her a safe journey, assuring us that we would see him in two weeks to remove the stiches and check her out. We wheeled Debbie triumphantly down to the main lobby and to the waiting car. Phil helped get her into the front seat, and I climbed in back so as to able to take care of her from there should the need arise.

It was 8:30 on a Saturday night when we pulled into the downtown CVS pharmacy with half a dozen prescriptions, three of which were controlled substances. The pharmacist took a look at the scripts and determined that they could not fill them there before closing time a half hour later. He quickly assessed the situation and the critical nature of the ask and made a call to a pharmacy in a suburb of Boston that was open twenty-four hours. They told him they could handle the request and he handed back our paperwork. I thanked him profusely and jumped back in the car for the trip home.

At about 9:30 p.m. we pulled into the Watertown CVS and I ran in with the prescriptions. Due to the controlled substances in the group, there would be about a one-hour wait for them to be able to fill them. I said go ahead and that we would stand by. I reported this back to Phil and Debbie, who were sitting in the car. We waited.

Phil was so great during this experience. While I waited in the CVS in case there was anything else needed, he waited with Debbie. At one point, she needed to use the bathroom and the two of them gingerly made their way into the store, picking up a couple of treats for the ride home while they were in there. They also listened to a street musician who was playing outside near the store parking lot. They did really well during the waiting time. Finally, at about 10:30, the prescriptions were filled and I jumped back in the car. We made the rest of the trip without incident and got back to our house at about 1:00 a.m. Sunday.

While the drama of Saturday unfolded at the hospital, our son Brian and his family of wife Liz, sons Patrick and Joe, and daughter Abigail all piled into their car and our car that I had driven up to Boston in and headed for our home in Winsted. There, they moved our bedroom from upstairs to downstairs, where the guest room was. This would allow us to have Debbie on just one level during her chemo treatments and recovery.

That move was quite a task for the family to do in just a few hours. They moved a Sleep Number bed downstairs with just two adults and then moved the queen bed that was in the guest room back upstairs. When we arrived home, the family was gone and the beds were all in place. We had to do nothing other than get Debbie from the car into bed. That was a really loving thing to do.

CHAPTER 6

Home

The next day we had a first meeting with the Visiting Nurses of Litchfield County. Two nurses arrived at the house, and there was an interview with Debbie to catch up on what had been done and what her physical and mental status were. Debbie was funny as she tried to show off what she could do, standing and sitting up; walking and talking; reaching and grabbing. The nurses were duly impressed by her capabilities at such an early stage of recovery. Debbie smiled.

From this interview, it was determined that Debbie would not need care every day and that they could come in once a week to check on her status. If we experienced any difficulties or had questions, we should contact them immediately. They gave Debbie some exercise tips and some recommendations for not getting too physical too fast. They noted that the wound was healing well and that Debbie had comfortable surroundings.

Debbie complained of headaches to the nurses. They said this was quite normal and that ice would help. She should take Tylenol if the pain persisted. There was also oxycodone in case the pain was too great.

The headache issue Debbie was having would continue for several weeks as her head healed from the surgery. It was apparently from the incision, not something inside. She complained of the pain often, and the only thing that seemed to alleviate it was an ice pack. She did not take the oxi, saying it was too dangerous.

Our living room had a very nice, large television and a comfortable couch. This became Debbie's happy place as her recovery continued. The VNA nurses came for visits and were encouraged by Debbie's improvements and lack of any noticeable ill effects from the surgery, other than the continuing headaches.

Debbie discovered Hallmark Channel at this time, and it became the staple for her to relax and get better. At this time, COVID was really affecting everyone throughout the country. We could have no visitors, so our friends were bringing food over and leaving it at the door. Debbie's sisters wanted to come and visit, but we were too afraid of the virus to even allow that. It was very isolating at a time when it would have been helpful to have visitors and family to be with us.

CHAPTER 7

Recuperation

For the next four weeks, Debbie rested and recuperated from the hospital ordeal. Though she wished she could go right back to being her old self, working and making pottery, she was forced to sit out much of what was going on around her.

Her head continued to hurt as it mended, and she seemed to constantly want ice on it. Her strength and ability to move around improved. Her drive to get better was phenomenal. Appetite improved, and we had what you might call a period of grace through the end of October and into November.

Just two weeks after getting home, the VNA released Debbie from further service. She was in really good shape and nearly back to normal in regard to getting around and managing her pain. She was a fighter and had shown the nurses she could do everything she wanted and needed to do on her own.

October 26th was the next scheduled visit back at Boston Medical Center to remove her stitches and get checked over by Dr. D. The night before, we spent a restless night in a fancy hotel down on the Boston Waterfront. The hotel was nearly empty due to COVID and no restaurants were open. I was able to order some food from the hotel kitchen, but I had to go down to the lobby to pick it up. We did not sleep much that night, and the morning came early with the fear of what would happen at the appointment.

Dr. D. met with us, and a very skilled nurse removed Debbie's stitches without too much pain. She asked Debbie to think of being in her favorite place, and we talked about our recent trip to Paris, France, the Christmas before all of this started.

Dr. D. said that Debbie's recovery was going very well and her incision was healing nicely. He then explained what would be happening next, which was that we would be switching Debbie's care over to Yale New Haven Hospital, under the care of neuro-oncologist Dr. B. He explained that he would like to continue to receive reports and copies of any MRI tests that Debbie would be receiving. He would follow up with us after a few months to see how things were going. We left relieved for having the stitches out but pensive regarding the next steps.

Later that same week, we had our first visit at Yale New Haven with Dr. B. Bloodwork was done, Debbie was checked over and questioned about her experience thus far. Then there was a lengthy discussion about the next steps.

Dr. B. explained that there was a positive finding in the pathology of the tumor. It was found to be methylated, which means that the typical treatments should be more effective than if it was not this type. There is a very strict protocol for treatment of glioblastoma multiform (GBM). This is done so that patients may be entered into clinical trials afterward. If the protocol is not followed, trials are not possible, according to clinical and insurance rules.

The tumor pathology was of great importance. Patients with methylated tumors have a greater lifespan record by almost double. Dr. B. explained that non-methylated tumor survival periods are a year to eighteen months, while methylated averages are often three to five years. There are outliers of course, with both shorter and longer lifespans.

He explained the protocol. Debbie would undergo radiation therapy every weekday for six weeks while also taking a daily oral chemotherapy regiment. Bloodwork would be done weekly to ensure that blood chemistry was still appropriate, since the chemo is known to drop platelet counts to dangerously low levels. Once this first radiation and chemo treatment was completed, there would be a four-week period for her body to rest and recuperate.

Then, a second phase of chemo would be started, which would be one week of chemo and three weeks of rest for six months. After that, MRI testing would be done every two months to watch for any recurrence of the tumor.

Dr. B. told us that we could utilize a radiation center close to home for the treatments, and he set up dialog with Dr. W., the radiation oncologist at a Torrington treatment center. We would begin that phase within the next two weeks.

We left the appointment with our heads spinning a bit from all the information. Yale New Haven is about an hour and fifteen minutes from our home. This trip became standard procedure for us on a monthly basis for the next several months and was often a time for us to discuss what we had heard and what we expected. On the way home from this first appointment, we talked a bit about the methylated finding and what that could mean to Debbie. She thought right away that she might be one of the outliers who lived past the normal ranges. In fact, I think she was certain of this. She has always been an outlier, beating odds in most of her other life experiences. Being the fighter she is, I tried to believe her.

Support from family kept coming as we worked through these early treatment preparations. One very sweet thing that happened about this time was when our daughter-in-law Liz contacted us and asked if we wanted to join them on a cruise. At first, I was shocked when she said it was in February, but she quickly added that it was to be in February 2022. She thought that would be some-thing we could keep in our minds and hope for the best. It turned out to be an important trigger for us to think about the future when the present sometimes seemed so bleak.

November 9th, 2020, was our first visit with Dr. W. at her office in Torrington. During that visit, more bloodwork was done to create a baseline for Debbie's levels. She was fitted with a special mask that would hold her head very rigid for the radiation treatments to come. The radiation would be aimed at a very specific area where the tumor had been located, and her head could not move during the treatments. Dr. W. explained more about the process and the schedule for treatments. They would be every weekday at around the same time, as much as possible.

On Thursday, November 10th, Debbie and I went to Lowe's to pick out an artificial Christmas tree. She has always loved everything about Christmas, and it was my plan to put up a tree early and enjoy it as long as we could. We brought home a very nice tree with built-in lights and a very realistic look. The next day, our oldest son, Aaron, and his youngest daughter, Meredith, came to visit for the weekend, knowing this was likely to be an emotional time when both Debbie and I could use family around. They wanted to be at our house when Debbie got home from her first treatment.

Friday, November 11th, we rose early to begin the oral chemo treatments. I gave Debbie a pill to reduce nau-sea, which was expected from the temozolomide that she would be taking. A half hour later, she received her first chemo treatment. We opted to do this every morning so that Debbie could be in bed during the first hour of treatment every day. This worked out well, and Debbie had few ill effects from the pills.

Later that day, we headed to the radiation treatment facility in Torrington for her first radiation. Aaron and Meredith remained at home. The treatment went fine, though Debbie was quite afraid at first. With COVID still rampant in our area, the treatment facility had strict rules about only having one or two people in the waiting room, so scheduling was tight and the room was very quiet. I had to wait in the waiting room while Debbie had her treatments. The did not take very long, and we were there each day for only about a half hour.

When we got home, Debbie was exhausted by the stress of the first treatment, and her head felt strange to her. Ice helped and she lay on the couch for the rest of the day. Aaron and Meredith surprised us by having the Christmas tree up and decorated when we got home. This cheered Debbie up immensely and the night was fairly peaceful.

That weekend, the chemo ritual continued and we got into a rhythm. Debbie was still not feeling much ill effect from the pills, though the nausea pill did cause some constipation. Her appetite diminished a bit, though, and finding food that she liked began to be a challenge.

Sunday, Aaron and Meredith left and we were on our own again, heading into the first full week of treatments.

First thing each morning was the chemo treatment, and then midday we headed to the radiation center. Debbie complained of some headaches, which Dr. W. explained could happen due to the radiation. What we did not realize for a while was that Debbie's scalp and hair were actually being burned by the radiation.

Debbie began to complain of a smell that made her feel very sick to her stomach. Food began to be an issue if the smell was strong. In fact, Debbie could not open the refrigerator without feeling very sick, so I took over all cooking and food preparation. She could not eat all foods that she used to enjoy. Often, I would prepare dinner and she would take one fork full and put it back, unable to finish even one bite. My new challenge was to find foods that she could eat. We found that macaroni and cheese was a good one and ice cream always worked. I tried other recipes to vary our diet a bit, but many times Debbie could not eat what was prepared. This went on through the entire six weeks of radiation, and Debbie lost quite a bit of weight during that time.

Our daily routine was very steady. Chemo, then radiation, then rest. Debbie's strength during this time was quite low, though her fighting spirit never wavered. We had few guests, as COVID was a great fear with Debbie's immune system so weakened by the treatments. Our friends continued to bring food, and some even had food kits shipped to us. Most times, poor Debbie could eat none of it. We tried each new recipe as it came into the house, but her smell and taste were so harshly affected by the treatments that she often could not eat a bite of it. Back to the mac and cheese or ice cream we went to in order to have something in her.

Each week Debbie had bloodwork to determine if her levels were still good enough to continue all the treatments. Each week the levels dropped a bit, but were still safe. Debbie made herself eat something substantial the night before each test, thinking that she had to keep going. She was very afraid that the chemo might have to be stopped or that an infusion of platelets might have to be given to keep it going.

One night, I walked into the bedroom to help her get ready for bed and she swooned, saying that she could not take the smell of me. I was quite devastated. I did not know what I could do to help and I did not know how I even smelled. It was a very low point for both of us. Her sense of smell had become a negative superpower, and it was hurting us both. I stayed away that night, and thankfully the next day was a little bit better. The things we both had to put up with during this treatment time were very hard for us. We had always been very close, and now I could not even be close enough to her to hold her or comfort her. I was nearly at my wits' end.

Four weeks into the treatments, her blood levels dropped markedly, and the decision was made to send Debbie to Yale New Haven for an infusion that would bring the levels up enough to keep going. To have to stop now would be very detrimental to the entire treatment plan. We made the trip to New Haven and her blood was checked again. It was found to be just high enough to not have to have the infusion. We headed back home and the next day we were back on track with both chemo and radiation.

Five weeks into the treatments, her bloodwork was very low again. There were only five more scheduled chemo days, and Doctor B. at Yale determined that the chemo could be stopped at that point without endangering the outcome of the treatment. Debbie would continue to have radiation, but no more chemo.

December 24th, was Debbie's last day of radiation treatments. She had done it. We had done it. Christmas came and went very quietly as Debbie recuperated from the very demanding protocol. We thanked God for the end of it. Debbie could rest a bit now.

For Christmas, we had not really thought much about gifts for each other. Debbie had heard me talking about some special western boots that kept showing up on my Facebook feed. One night, she told me to order them for my Christmas present and I did. They were shipped to the house about a week before Christmas, and she made me wait to open them Christmas morning. That was sweet and I still cherish those boots.

For her gift, I had a hard time thinking of something that would be meaningful in these times. It finally came to me, and I spent a morning up in my woodshop cutting out and staining a sign that we could put up prominently in our living room where she would see it every day. It simply said "OUTLIER" and she loved it. I think she loved me for thinking of it too. In those days, it was not always easy for me to show my support for her so strongly believing in her ability to beat the odds with this disease.

That Christmas was a time when I struggled with the difference between positive thinking and denial. While I truly wanted Debbie to be positive and keep fighting, I also felt that the statistics and history of GBM were so strong that in my own mind I thought she should be more realistic. This philosophical struggle was a constant issue with me throughout our experience with GBM. Over the past three years, I have come to realize that it does not matter what I think about it; it matters what Debbie thinks about it. Her right is to be positively thinking up to and through the point that I might feel is denial. That was her choice to make, not mine. And I must deal with it in my own way, typically through talking with other people aside from us.

2020 ended quietly. The drama of our lives since September 26th was something we never saw coming. Debbie had seemed just fine prior to the seizures, though she had been having headaches all summer. She had thought those were just stress headaches caused by the demands of running the transfer station and keeping her employees safe during the height of COVID. Now, we understood that the headaches had been a sign of the disease sneaking up on her. These past three months were a shock to both of us and we hoped the worst was behind us.

CHAPTER 8

January through March 2021 – Recuperation

Once the holidays were through, Debbie needed some real rest and recuperation to build up her muscles and energy again. Lying on the couch or in beds for three months had not helped her muscle tone or stamina and she needed to feel better. Her fighting spirit began to pick up again. During that month, she thought more and more about getting back to work, though her energy would not allow it yet. She moved around the house and pushed herself to do some things to work her tired muscles. We even took a ride to RRDD1, where she was still the administrator, though the team had really picked up the slack while she was out of action. Tears were shed by Debbie and the crew as we met them and Debbie walked around the office a bit to greet those who were working.

Debbie met with her general practitioner, Dr. S., during the first week of the month and got a thorough check-up. Dr. S. was pleased with the healing and recommended that Debbie have vaccines to prevent any flu or COVID problems over the coming months. Debbie had the shots. They also discussed Debbie having a colonoscopy soon, as she had never had one. I was skeptical of the need for it, but Dr. S. advised it strongly, even in the current situation. We left with a positive attitude with hopes for continued improvements.

Later in the month, Debbie had an MRI at Yale to determine what effects the radiation had on the tumor area. Then we met with Dr. W. a few days later to go over the results. Dr. W. told us the radiation had done its job and the area appeared quite clear. She explained that the headaches and smell issues should not be a factor going forward, and we were happy with that. She bid us good luck with the upcoming second phase of treatments that would not include radiation, just chemotherapy.

The next few weeks were a time of ongoing improvements, and Debbie began to feel a bit like her old self again. She longed to get back to normal, working and traveling as we always had. Her spirits were good and her positive attitude surprised all who encountered her.

In mid-February, the second phase of chemotherapy was to begin. On February 15th, Debbie started temozolomide treatments on a one week out of every four weeks basis. During treatment weeks, we went through the same process as we had during the previous treatments. Anti-nausea medicine, then TMZ a half hour later. This new schedule was much easier on her body. She was feeling all right for the first two days and then would begin to feel the side effects of tiredness and even some taste and smell issues. Luckily, these symptoms abated quickly once the treatments were done. By mid-week of the week following the treatments, she was back to normal.

In early March, we had another visit to Yale with Dr. B. He reviewed the results of the first treatments of this new phase and bloodwork was done to check on Debbie's levels. Everything looked good for continuing the treatments.

During March, we both got a bit of spring fever going. In 2020 we had received a very small fishing boat from my friend Griff, and we had really enjoyed getting out into the local ponds for some fishing. Debbie loved to fish, as long as I put the worms on her hook. Her look of delight and excitement when she got a little fish on the end of her line was wonderful. I loved taking her out, and I think she enjoyed the fishing possibly even more than I did. She certainly was better at it than me, catching far more little fish than I did.

We decided that we would definitely go fishing more this year, and plans began to turn into action as I bought some antique fishing gear that I thought might be interesting to use in our local ponds.

Debbie also was really wanting to be back at work again. We went to the office a few times, me driving of course, and she picked up some things to be worked on at home. She perked up more and more as she thought about things other than her illness and treatments.

CHAPTER 9

April through June – Back to Normal

Debbie's goal was to get back to normal. She looked around at friends and family for cancer role models and found many who had cancer and beat it. She believed she was an outlier and would beat GBM too. Regardless of what doctors or I said, she knew she would do it. I tried my best not to squelch this, though it was very hard for me when I heard doctors and others speak about the probabilities. This was to be an ongoing dilemma for me as her husband and also care giver. It took until much later in the process for me to give up trying to bring in some reality to the conversations. I am sorry now that I did not give in much earlier, though it still would have been difficult knowing what I knew. Thinking about this now, I believe there is NO difference between positive thinking and denial in this case, and that the patient has every right to use either of those emotions to keep themselves going. Every right.

On April 16th, Debbie went back to work full time. During the weeks she had treatments, we just went in a little later to the office. I drove her, since it was not allowed for her to drive for six months after surgery for seizures. Luckily, due to COVID, I had been working from home since we came back from Boston, and I could work around taking her to the office and medical procedures.

Just after Debbie got back to work, I convinced her that we should buy a bigger fishing boat. We found a beautiful fourteen-footer that a man nearby was selling and we went to see it. We both loved it and we bought it right away. It had a trailer and many accessories and was all we would need for our fishing excursions to the lakes throughout Northwest Connecticut. I was so excited as we towed it home that first day. It ended up being something we both enjoyed numerous times in the coming months.

Later that month, I also sold my old Honda motorcycle. We had not ridden it for a couple of years, since a fall took some of the joy out of it, though that is another story. I knew that with Debbie's condition, we would never ride it again, so I wanted to sell it before it rotted in our barn. A man in Florida bought it and it was picked up by a friend of his. He loved Honda 750s, and I knew it was going to a good home. The money we got from it bought some more goodies for our new boat and fishing too. So, it was really a win-win for us.

April was also when Debbie began to get back into her pottery. She had not been able to work with clay for several months and was so happy to get back to it. She continued making pots and helping at the studio where she was part owner throughout the coming years. She was very prolific in what she produced and sold for the studio. She loved craft fairs, too, and we went to many even after she had been sick.

May came and went without major incident. Debbie grew stronger now that she was back at work and talked more about doing other things like traveling and seeing the grandkids. Treatments continued. For Memorial Day, we took our first family trip since the surgery. We visited Debbie's brother, Eddie, at his campsite in the Poconos. Eddie and his wife Joanie had purchased it the previous fall and were proud to have a family visit. Debbie's other sisters visited that weekend as well. There was an impromptu candle ceremony in remembrance of their sister Terri, who had passed away in March of the previous year. It was a special weekend with some tears, some great stories, and lots of love. Debbie's siblings were quite shocked that Debbie's condition had improved so greatly since last they saw her. It was a very positive experience for everyone.

Debbie showed me so often the power of positive thinking. She did not let even the toughest problems stop her from doing what she wanted to do. At this point,

Debbie was back to work and back to making pottery. She was visiting family and planning for the future. She was even helping out with the local ambulance association where she had been a volunteer EMT for so many years. She could no longer go on ambulance calls, but she did about everything else. She had been treasurer for several years and jumped back in to help with that in any way she could. She helped with bookkeeping on their pension plan and counselled current officers on issues of finance. There was little that she would not do in order to make herself feel back to normal.

The treatments were going well to this point, so in June we broached the subject of travel with Dr. B. Our son Aaron, who is a colonel in the Marine Corps, was stationed at Twenty-Nine Palms in the desert of California. Our other son Brian, who is an education consultant and living in Boston, was planning a trip out to visit Aaron's family and travel together to Flagstaff, AZ, for a family vacation. Debbie wanted to go too. We spoke with Dr. B. about it, and he determined that we could move the treatment scheduled for that same two-week period to a time after we returned without negative results. We were quite thrilled, and plans were made, ending June on a very high note.

CHAPTER 10

July through October – Travel and Status Quo

Summer was upon us, and Debbie was feeling better and better. We flew out to California on July 3rd, meeting our son at the airport in Palm Springs. He drove us up through the desert valleys to Twenty-Nine Palms, a small desert town in which one of the Marine Corps' most important training grounds exists. Though desolate, the desert was quite beautiful. The heat was immense, and the change from Connecticut climate was great. It was great to reach the camp and see where Aaron and his family were living. Their house was in a very nicely manicured neighborhood with southwest-styled homes and almost no grass. We could not get over how different it was from home.

The next day, we packed everything in the cars and headed out further into the desert and up to Flagstaff, Arizona. The boys (Aaron and Brian) had rented an entire house for our weeklong stay in Flagstaff. With all the kids and grandkids, plus Debbie and me, there were twelve of us there, and there was plenty of room.

The rental house was our base of operations for the next few days. We traveled up to see the Grand Canyon one day. The immensity of it was stunning. Debbie and I had been there a couple of years before in the late winter, so the summer foliage and scenery were all new to us too. Debbie was well enough by this time to even do some mild hiking, so we all walked to the rim and checked out several lookout points. It was so good to be with the whole family and do something with them that was quite normal. My heart swelled with joy to see Debbie with the grandkids. They tend to swarm her and love touching and hugging her, so this was a very special day.

Another day we headed for Sonoma, a small valley town south of Flagstaff that is known for its canyons and artsy vibe. Debbie and I splurged for a couple of jeeps to take us all into the back country for a canyon tour. The jeeps crawled over creek beds and rocks too large for anything but off-road vehicles. We bounced our way down the trails, strapped into the jeeps with five-point harnesses, laughing and gasping all the way. We reached the remnants of a small cabin way back in the canyon and stopped for a look. One of our best ever family photos was taken that day and everyone was smiling. Such memories are so important in normal times, so very special in limited times.

After a couple more days in Flagstaff, the entire family headed out. Aaron's family, Debbie, and I headed back to Twenty-Nine Palms. Brian and his family headed for Las Vegas and then on a trip home to Boston. We stayed in California for several more days before heading home. This trip proved that Debbie was indeed fit for travel and most normal activities again.

Upon arriving back in Connecticut, it was time for Debbie's last round of chemo. This went uneventfully and she was done.

In August, the local Firemen's Carnival was held in the last week of August. Debbie wanted to participate, so she helped with ticket sales for rides, and I helped in the Bingo tent. It felt great for us to be back out volunteering together again. Even with all the surgery, chemo, and radiation on her poor brain, Debbie was still able to think like she always did. She was one of the smartest people I ever knew, and she could balance several projects at the same time. Back during the early stages of treatment and recovery, I had worried that she might be affected negatively in that regard, but by this time in August it was obvious that was not the case. Debbie was normal again.

For Labor Day, we went back up to Eddie's campsite. This time, we were tempted to purchase a camper! He had just moved from his original site to a spot by the camp pond and his old site, along with a beautiful camper, was for sale. We headed up to look at it. It was a nice spot and a great camper, a larger fifth-wheel style camper. We thought hard about it for an hour back at Eddie's site. We were conflicted because the camp is about three hours from our home, and we were not sure how often we could get there, especially with all the other things we like to do. But it was a nice dream. Thankfully, within an hour, friends stopped by Eddie's camper and told us they had put in an offer. Whew, we dodged a bullet on that one. The issue had been decided for us. News came back shortly that the offer was accepted and the friends had their camper. Things certainly move fast sometimes.

Once we got back home, September rolled through without further incidents. Debbie, finally done with all the treatments, continued to get back to normal. The doctors told us that because Debbie had done all of the required treatments and was doing well, there was nothing left to do but have an MRI every two months to watch for changes. They also told us that she would be an excellent candidate for clinical trials of new treatments if the situation changed in the future.

Things were good for us as we marked the one-year anniversary of Debbie's seizure at Brian's house. September 26th came and went without issue. Our day-to-day life changed into week-to-week at this point. We were no longer checking the calendar every day for the next appointment or treatment. We were not keeping track of every pill and every hour for more pills. Debbie's attitude was to be who she had always been and do whatever she wanted to do. Work was good at RRDD1 and she was driving there on her own again. She was making pottery in the studio. She was helping at the ambulance headquarters.

I was working normal hours, still from home at this point. My day-to-day life changed back to my normal interests too. We fished when we could make time. I played golf with friends. I was active in our local Elks Lodge. Debbie, too, was active in the lodge as she was a member and had been through the same officer positions I had been in over the years. Our Elks friends were like family for us too. Since the boys lived far away, the Elks became our second family. Our friends there were close and helpful. At this time, we did not know just how helpful they would be to us someday. We found that out later.

CHAPTER 11

October through December – Situation Normal

The next three months were so normal it is hard to look back on them now and think of anything special that happened. We worked. We attended Elks events. One of those was the annual Halloween party, at which I won for the scariest costume. We dressed up as an angel, Debbie of course, and a devil, me of course. It was hysterical and we had a blast just like old times.

Debbie made pottery and sold it at several craft fairs with her fellow studio friends. Her work took on a new, more intense look. Each piece seemed to be made with a purpose. She was known for her organic style, especially with the large leaf platters that were made by taking leaves she had gathered and pressing them into the soft clay. She had a way of curling the edges to give them an appearance of life itself and then glazing them with soft greens and browns. They were beautiful and everybody loved them. She also made some crazy-looking bowls, or vases, that came up like a bowl but had waves and crinkles toward the top. People could not guess how she made these and they looked wild. She also loved making small vessels and plates for decoration or in any ways people could imagine. All were very organic and special. Friends at the studio always admitted to me that Debbie sold the most pottery at sales and in the studio gallery. I don't know why, but people just liked it.

As Christmas came closer, you could hardly tell, because we had the tree still up from the year before. We never took it down. Often, people remarked about how beautiful it looked, and Debbie just loved to sit and look at it. She loved Christmas time more than anyone I knew. It made her feel good, I guess, because she was such a giving person anyway. The Hallmark Channel, with its constant run of Christmas movies, was on all the time. We loved to sit and watch them, and even teared up a bit during the ones that were based on a loss in the family. That was a good Christmas season, and we were very thankful that Debbie was doing so well.

The week between Christmas and New Year's was spent with the family and we had a great time. We had some pretty special gifts for everyone, and it felt good to be able to give them. Both Debbie and I were working and times were good. Finances were good. Worries did not creep into our heads too much that season.

CHAPTER 12

January through March 2022 – The Cruise

As January came in, cold and clear, we prepared for another MRI. These MRI days were challenging because first we planned on them and thought about them for a week in advance. Then, the day of the MRI, we timed our trip to arrive at Yale New Haven about fifteen minutes before Debbie was to report to the radiology center so we would not be waiting too long. Then, once we got to the hospital, we had to check in and make our way to the waiting room. Debbie's MRIs were complex in that she needed one with no contrast and then one with contrast created by an intravenous injection of special die. The entire procedure took about an hour. Once that was done and she got dressed again, we either headed right for Dr.

B.'s office or down for a snack, depending upon the time between appointments.

Over the past year, we had gotten used to this routine. Dr. B. always checked Debbie out first and then walked through the MRI screens with us, each time showing us how there was no change from the last pictures. It got to be a strange joke where Debbie and I poked fun at the report, saying, "Well, no change this time." We began both to believe there would never be a change and the MRIs could become more and more distant. We prayed this would happen. Even I started to think maybe Debbie could be the first person to actually beat this disease. She certainly was determined enough to do it.

The rest of January was normal for this time of year. Work, eat, rest, work, eat, rest. It got dark so early that the days seemed short and the nights really long unless we went to bed early. Hallmark movies kept us occupied.

February came and suddenly here was the cruise we said yes to so long ago in bad times. We excitedly flew down to Florida a day early and enjoyed the summer-like heat. The cruise was a wonderful break in the routine of winter. Debbie and I were feeling like we had perhaps beaten something very bad and this was a celebration of that feat. The seas were calm and the islands beautiful. It was a perfect time.

On the cruise, Debbie let me buy another watch for my collection of nice watches. It was exciting to go through the process of learning about the watches in a short luncheon seminar, then going to the jewelry shop onboard ship to look at the fine selection. I chose one that suited our taste and it was mine.

On the last island we visited, we went to another jewelry shop at the pier. This was on the island of St. Kitts, which was our favorite stop on the cruise. We had spent the sunny afternoon on a beach overlooking a windjammer ship in the harbor. It was a special day. We entered the jewelry shop with a pseudo-cavalier attitude, just looking of course. We happened across a beautiful set of bejeweled finger ring and earrings. They were quite spectacular and expensive by our standards. I looked Debbie in the eyes and said we should get them. She hesitated, and I knew it was because she did not know for how long she would wear these gifts. I did not hesitate. "We should get them if you like them." I believe you cannot stop buying beautiful gifts for your favorite person, just because time may be limited. We bought them and Debbie loved them forever.

This cruise was an important time for us and for Brian, Liz, and the grandkids. We were able to share moments with them away from home that could not be duplicated at home. Travel had always meant a lot to Debbie and me, and this trip was a very special one. We arrived back home refreshed and ready to continue the fight, though at that time it did not seem like much of a fight. These were fine times.

Soon, we were in March. The month flew by and suddenly we were celebrating Debbie's birthday. Debbie turned sixty-five on March 30th. It was a big day, and I knew she was celebrating many things. Because Debbie turned sixty-five, her driver's license needed to be renewed. Since she was driving again, this was important and we renewed it. I never told her, but I only renewed it for one year this time. I just could not force myself to renew for five years. I felt guilty about that for a time, but I knew it was probably the right decision, and anyway, we could renew it again the next year.

CHAPTER 13

April through July –
Travel and Leisure

In April, we decided that we needed another trip and we began to plan. Our oldest granddaughter, Ceceilia, was to graduate from high school in June, in Twenty-nine Palms. We decided to attend it, and as an added bonus we would attend Aaron's change of command ceremony where he would transfer the reigns of command over to a new colonel. He had finished his tour there as leader of the Marine Corp Logistics School and would be heading back to the east coast to work at the Pentagon.

April was also an important time for me. I had decided that it was a good time for me to retire from my company. I had worked for the same company for forty-three years.

The company had just been sold to a major competitor, the second sale in three years. I was exhausted by the changes happening in that sphere of my life. I was out of shape, weighing in at two-hundred twenty-two pounds, drinking too much, and not feeling great about my own health. My department was responsible for reporting the month-to-month sales figures in every conceivable way, and it was becoming more and more difficult to keep up with the changes. At the same time, my department's reports meant less to the new company, and I did not even really know to whom I was reporting. It was time to go.

So, on April 27th, I retired from my position. A retirement party happened in the cafeteria at work, and many friends from the old company were there. There was cake and a few gifts, and I was quite misty-eyed to be leaving after so many good years and hard work.

To celebrate, Debbie and her best friend Colleen had arranged a trip to Pennsylvania to see a show by their favorite musician, Peter Noone. We traveled with Colleen by car down to Jim Thorpe, a quaint little town in the hills of eastern PA. The town is full of local history, including the tale of the Molly McGuires, who were a group of Irish coal miners who fought with the local mine owners to make a better life for the miners. The fight was quite brutal at times, and several of the Molly McGuire members were arrested, imprisoned, and hanged in the local jail in town. The story was a powerful one, and as I walked through the town the morning after we arrived, I felt the presence of these fighters. Perhaps in some way, I felt a kinship with them in their fight for a better life.

Later, we thoroughly enjoyed the show put on by Peter Noone, and I was surprised to find out that Debbie and Colleen had paid for my membership of his fan club. We got special treatment before the show and got to meet with Peter after the band's warm-up. Peter was up on stage and answered questions from the fan club members who were there. Unbeknownst to me, Debbie had slipped him a note that I had just retired and was the newest member of the club. He read it onstage and bid me good luck in front of everyone. I was quite embarrassed and thrilled at the same time.

On the way home from the concert trip, Debbie was feeling quite poorly. She was very tired and felt achy all over. Two days later, I received a text from my friend who had thrown the party at work for me. She was beside herself. She found out she and another friend who was there tested positive for COVID, and I may have contracted it as well. Unbelievable! I had worked from home for two years in order to avoid COVID. Now, on my last day of work for the company, I got it. We tested immediately and found that indeed we, too, had COVID. I had to contact Colleen and some other folks who I had been around over the past week to let them know. Luckily, Colleen and the others were clear. Debbie and I spent the next several days watching Hallmark and resting. Our case was mild and we had few symptoms. It was a bit of a wakeup call for us, though. We had to watch out, because a serious illness could affect Debbie more now than before her illness.

I had set a goal for myself to get healthier by the end of my first year of retirement. Enough of the sitting around. I began walking through town, trying every day to walk a little farther. Soon, I was walking over two miles each day and feeling better about myself. I was still drinking too much, but I figured that would work out later. I think in the back of my mind I had a good reason to drink. Alcohol dulled the feeling of loss that I was starting to feel at times. So, my walking counteracted my drinking. That made sense to me.

In May, Debbie was focused on producing more pottery for upcoming shows and this became her emphasis again for a while. She produced some beautiful pieces in that time. We also had a special amateur radio event focused on the town's two-hundred-fiftieth anniversary. We applied for a special event callsign and operated radios a lot during the week leading up to the anniversary celebration. We had over two-hundred-fifty contacts and set up an operating radio at the celebration event. Our lives had come back to doing the things we loved and not just the things we had to do, for work or for Debbie's cancer.

June 6th, on my sixty-sixth birthday, we took off from Hartford for California again. Megan picked us up at Palm Springs airport, and we took that familiar ride up through the desert valleys to Twenty-nine Palms. This time the trip was centered in that area exclusively. Debbie and I stayed in a hotel on base for the first two nights, as the house was being packed up for the big move. Megan's parents, Joan and Michael, were in town, too, for Ceceilia's graduation. Mike and Joan had to leave after graduation, and we remained for the change of command later in that week. After the graduation ceremony, we moved to a very special old motor inn in Joshua Tree, the tiny town just west of Twenty-nine Palms. We moved there because Aaron, Megan, and the girls finished their pack out of the house and moved off base to a weekly rental in Josua Tree, just up the hill from our hotel.

The Joshua Tree Inn was famous, mostly for the fact it had been the hangout for music stars back in the 1970s. Most famous of those was Graham Parsons, who had written many spacy country songs at that time and was friends with all the top bands from everywhere. He used to bring his friends up to Joshua Tree to get away from the pressures of Los Angeles and to wander through Joshua Tree National Park. One night, Graham Parsons died in one of the rooms of that little inn and it became a famous landmark. In fact, there was a little shrine in the courtyard of the inn that had fresh deposits from fans who still came to visit just because of Graham's passing there.

There was a very spiritual feeling in the courtyard and throughout the inn. Both Debbie and I loved being there, and it felt like there was energy flowing through us. When I could help myself no longer, I went into the office to share my strange feeling with the girls behind the counter. I felt a little funny mentioning it, but they both smiled broadly and said back, "Why do you think we work here?" They explained that there was a local company that tracked "vortex" activity in the area, and they had determined there was one such vortex in the courtyard. Believe it, or don't, we both felt strange vibrations from that place and remembered it ever after.

While at Joshua Tree, we visited the park with Aaron and Megan and even took a drive out into it on our own a time or two. The park is a vast high desert with one of the strangest trees to be found anywhere, the Joshua Tree. It is about the size of a large bush or shrub and is shaped a bit like a cactus. The trees were all over the park, and it was a beautiful and serene place.

We also enjoyed some time up at the rental house. There was a pool in the backyard, and Debbie swam for the first time since being in the hospital. She loved it and got so brave that Aaron and Megan both jumped in the pool to make sure she did not overdo it. I think it scared and delighted them that Debbie enjoyed it so. They were both relieved, though, when Debbie had enough and got out to sit on the lounge chairs to get some sun. It was a great time.

The change of command ceremony came later in the week, just the day before we all had to leave. It was exciting to see Aaron transfer the flag from him to the new commanding officer. We were so proud of him and his boss, the general, explained to all that Aaron had done an outstanding job. Pictures were taken and hands were shaken. After the celebration we headed back to the rental house for a special dinner and relaxed into the evening. The next morning we headed down to Palm Springs to stay one night before the plane trip home. Aaron, Megan, and the girls headed out on their long journey back east. It had been a great trip.

Once home, Debbie and I settled back into our summer routine. We traveled a couple of times over the next few weeks, to Pennsylvania and to Boston to visit family in both places. I continued my walking every day and working outside a bit. I was beginning to lose weight, and I set a goal to be under two-hundred pounds by Christmas.

On July 25th, we had another MRI day in New Haven. Once again, we were relieved to hear Dr. B. tell us "No changes, Debbie. You are doing great!" The words we loved to hear.

CHAPTER 14

August through October – Summertime Fades

During August, Debbie continued to build pottery stock for a very busy schedule of craft fairs in the fall. She planned on attending seven different shows, an aggressive plan for sure. Her pottery was getting more and more stylized, and the organic nature of it was stunning.

While Debbie was definitely having a powerful burst of energy and productivity during this time, I was not quite sure where I was headed. I was very happy to not be working anymore, but I was not feeling really comfortable in my skin. I was taking some time off, I guess, to figure out what I wanted to do. I was drinking more and more often. Debbie expressed concern a few times, but generally left me alone about it. She had not been able to drink since the first seizure and was taking anti-seizure medication that prohibited any alcohol consumption. But I was finding more reasons to enjoy alcohol, and it had turned from beer to whiskey. I did not know it at the time, but I was headed for trouble.

One day, late in August, we attended the Van Gogh traveling exhibit in Hartford. It was very moving. We both had loved his work before, and the historical information shared in the show added to our feelings. The three-dimensional aspect of the show was overpowering. There was a great hall of vast projected images of his work that moved and flowed as patrons watched. We sat on a bench for quite some time and took it in. Both of us were quite speechless by the end. The beauty and sadness of his work remained with us long after we were finished.

The Firemen's Carnival was that weekend and we once again worked at it. Debbie enjoyed selling the tickets to all the townspeople, especially ones she knew. I had a great time working in the bingo booth, even calling bingo for a while. It felt good to volunteer for such an important local organization.

For a long time, I had thought about doing some writing. When the local college listed a class on American Literature from 1840 to present day, I figured that would be a nice way to jump-start my writing spirit. I signed up for the class and it began in early September. Every Tuesday and Thursday, I walked to the college with my books in my backpack and attended the classes. I was old enough to be the grandparent of the rest of the students, and it gave me a chance to share some of my views and ideas with some very bright kids. We became quite close as we critiqued works from civil war times to the present authors. We wrote papers and critical essays. It got my creative juices flowing.

Debbie had a desire to get her teeth cleaned and have a checkup, so we scheduled that and she went to our dentist of many years. She was cleared with no new cavities and healthy gums. Then, she decided that she needed new glasses. She scheduled an eye exam and found out that her eyes had improved over the past couple of years, and there was no damage from the surgery to her peripheral vision, as had been feared by the doctors in Boston. She got her new glasses and happily announced to anyone who would listen that her eyes were great.

In late September, we were invited to attend the wedding of our niece's oldest son, to be held in Pennsylvania near Allentown. The whole family was in for this wedding and it was time for celebration. The day before the wedding, we stopped in Springbrook and stayed at the old homestead, as did quite a few other traveling family members. A pre-wedding party was bound to break out that night, so I picked up some beer and a quart of Jameson whiskey, to be shared by guests.

That night as family arrived at the house, festivities began and drinks flowed freely. Debbie was busy with other family and I was sitting at the table with my nephew.

It turned out that everyone had brought their own favorites to drink. Without really noticing it, my whiskey glass was never empty. I was just drinking it with ice, so it went down too easy. The party got more and more fun and loud. I was having a great time. I did not realize I finished that whole bottle!

The next morning, I slept pretty late and had a strange dream. I dreamed that since I was no longer needed at the office, I was no longer needed anywhere. I dreamed that I could die anytime and it would matter to nobody. I had become unnecessary. With a start, I woke up. Still feeling kind of funky, I just lay there for a little while. Debbie woke up next to me and asked how I was feeling. I said all right but was not really sure. She said, "I woke up around 1:30 and you were not in bed. I looked around the house and you were not here. I found the front door open and looked outside to find you sitting on the front porch swing. I asked you what you were doing and you said you were just talking with your friends."

I was quite shocked by this as I remembered none of it. She asked if I realized I had drunk the whole bottle of whiskey and I answered that I did not know that. The dream came back to me and I told her about it. She suggested that I have no alcohol for a while and I had to agree.

The rest of that day was horrible. I had to drive about two hours to get us to the wedding, and the entire time I was just trying to keep steady and in the moment. It was a tough drive. We were very quiet during the ride, and I thought back to that dream and what it meant. I began to realize that it was a strong sign that my life was in disorder. I had not separated myself from my job well enough toward the end of my career. Instead of being a man who ran reports and managed a team, I had been a manager and report writer who was a man only in off hours. I realized how wrong I was to think that way. Debbie needed me, though lately she had not seemed to need me like she did when I was taking care of her after her surgery. Things were starting to come together for me as we pulled into the hotel where we stayed for the wedding.

I laid down on the bed and almost fell asleep, but Debbie pushed me to get up and get moving. We went to the wedding and the reception afterward where I was still feeling a bit sheepish about the party and the dream. The family was very friendly and nothing was said about it. The reception was non-alcoholic anyway, so that was helpful. We celebrated and enjoyed the time with all the family around.

That night, I collapsed into bed and slept very soundly. The next day, Debbie and I talked more about the incident, and I determined that I would not drink alcohol for a while. I felt stronger making the decision. I also felt a new feeling of purpose after that dream. I realized that Debbie needed me and was concerned for my wellbeing. Tough times might be coming, and I would need to have my wits about me.

We headed home from the weekend with some new ideas and cherished each other a little bit more. It was somehow positive to have gone through it, though I'm not sure I recommend the exact process I went through.

The second weekend in October was the most prestigious craft fair of the season at Berkshire Botanical. We headed up the day before the show to set up the booth. The show went well and we were off and running on our fall craft tour.

After another short trip to Boston in mid-October, we headed to Yale for another MRI. After going through the normal ritual, Debbie and I waited in the office for Dr. B. to come in. We were told that one of his associates would be joining us first to go over the checkup and MRI results and then Dr. B. would join at the end. We waited a bit and there was a quiet knock on the door. Dr. B. came into the office and sat down. He went through the routine dexterity tests with Debbie and turned to the computer to go over the MRI results. "Debbie, there has been a change." The words stung us both with an unexpected clenching of the gut. "A change?"

Dr. B. showed the slides comparing the July MRI with the October MRI, and there was a definite change in the configuration of the right temporal lobe. A shadow appeared where there had been nothing before. The shading indicated that there was a slight growth along with traces of something moving out from the same area as the original tumor. The tumor was back. Our illusion of beating the disease was suddenly ripped to shreds.

Dr. B. went on to say that more time would be needed to determine exactly what was happening, but it appeared something was changing. There was nothing to do at this point except wait until the next MRI in December. At that time, we would determine the best options to go forward.

Our ride home that night was very long, very quiet, and a bit tearful. Debbie was silent for most of the trip, processing what this could mean. She was also fighting mad, because she had believed she was going to beat this so much that she could not accept this blow.

The next day, we continued on. We both knew something was up, but we did not want to think about it. Later that week, we took a previously scheduled ride on a steam train in Essex, CT. It was enjoyable, and I think we started cherishing any times like these we would have together.

CHAPTER 15

November through December – Treading Water

On November 4th, we attended a seminar put on by Hartford Healthcare. It was focused on brain tumors, and GBM was the primary focus. We heard speakers discussing the latest treatment techniques and statistics of the various forms of brain tumors. GBM was the most destructive and least treatable type. After the presentations and lunch, there was a breakout session for patients and for caregivers. During this, those people shared their background and stories, along with some fears. It was the first time Debbie and I had been to anything like it. Debbie reported back to me that she was reassured during her session that the doctors and cancer team would be fighting for her and that she should not think about statistics in general, that she is her own statistic. This was reiterated during the final session of the day. Every patient is their own statistic and should not allow themselves to be affected by the numbers. It was an important conference for us and gave us some new tools to work with when the options came up in December.

Within the next couple of weeks, we also bought a new car. Our Buick Verano had been a pretty good car, but we felt that if we needed to be certain of transportation, it was time for a new one. Thankfully, Debbie picked out a Buick Encore that was a small SUV and sat a bit higher than the Verano. It was much easier to get in and out of it, and it would hold a lot more stuff if need be. Having a hatchback instead of a trunk turned out to be a very important improvement.

Debbie had a couple of craft fairs in November and these went well. She was driven now to sell as much as she could to support the studio. She was driven now to do everything. She was still fighting mad about the change and was determined to keep moving.

For Thanksgiving we went to Brian's vacation house in New Hampshire and had a very nice time with the family. Debbie did not let the worry of change control her, and we enjoyed being with the grandkids any time we could.

In mid-December, we were invited to our nephew Bill's wedding. It was to be held in Austin, Texas, and several of the family planned to attend. We flew out two days before. Aaron and Megan came, too, and Brian and Liz flew out. We were in separate hotels, so we linked up for various meals and functions. It was a special weekend and we enjoyed Austin very much.

At the wedding, we were scattered throughout the great hall that Bill and Sameen had rented, meeting and greeting friends and family and other guests we had not known before. As we found our assigned dinner seats and sat with the boys, some of us were aware that Debbie was not her usual self. She was saying some things that were a bit out of character and stared off into space sometimes. Several of us noticed and began watching her a little closer. Something was off, but we could not quite put our fingers on it. It was mentioned a few times between several of us. She did all right for the rest of the night, but we kept an eye on her.

The weekend ended peacefully and we made our way back home. A few days later was Debbie's next scheduled MRI. We made our way to New Haven and passed through the normal routine. After getting dressed from the test, Debbie and I headed up to Dr. B.'s office for the follow-up appointment.

Dr. B. knocked quietly on the examination room door and entered. He sat down as always and asked how things had been going and if we had noticed any changes in feeling or behavior since the last appointment. Debbie and I explained what we could as Dr. B. listened and nodded. He turned to the computer screens and said, "Let's take a look at the results."

On the screen were comparison shots of the October MRI and that day's MRI. There was a marked difference between the two. The tumor had grown substantially and more toward the center than just around the outside of the brain. There were little trails going out from it toward the back. It was back and big again.

Dr. B. said, "It is time for us to discuss the options." He went on to explain that Debbie was an excellent candidate for a drug trial that was taking place at the time. This new drug was showing some signs of being able to help the body's own immune system identify the cancer cells and go after them. It was a new kind of immunotherapy that had shown positive results with some other cancers and was now being tested for GBM.

He went on to explain that in order to be part of the trial, the current tumor had to be removed and Debbie had to be cleared medically and physically to continue it. This would mean surgery again. The other options were to possibly try chemo again or to do nothing.

Given the options and the possibility of being part of a trial that could cure the cancer, Debbie quickly opted for that procedure. Dr. B. agreed. He explained that the trial had other requirements, such as having another MRI in January, just before the surgery, and having one trial infusion of the new drug a week or so before the surgery to see if it has any effect before surgery.

We agreed with these provisions and Dr. B. had us sign a release to begin the process. We left the appointment nervous but hopeful that this may be what Debbie needed in order to beat the cancer. There was really no other option except to give in, and Debbie was never into that scenario.

Christmas was celebrated at Brian and Liz's New Hampshire lodge. Aaron, Megan, and the girls all came up for the week as well. But before we went there, we needed to head to my mother's house in Canisteo, New York for a couple of days to celebrate Christmas morning with them. They were heading to Florida just a few days after Christmas, and we would not see them for months if we did not make this trip. It was a whirlwind trip, but we did not want to miss the opportunity, since Debbie would likely not be able to travel for a while after the next surgery.

The time with my mother was nice, though very short. We had an enjoyable Christmas Eve dinner with her and my stepfather Don. We woke up on Christmas to a frosty morning and headed out on the road to get back to our house for one night and then up to New Hampshire.

The rest of the week between Christmas and New Year's was with our boys and their family, and we made the most of it. I had made it through three months without drinking, other than a couple of beers in Austin. I was feeling healthier than I had in a long time. My weight was down to about one-hundred-ninety pounds, beating my goal of weighing below two-hundred pounds.

Debbie and the grandkids cuddled and giggled through much of the week. We had some quiet times, but mostly did not think or talk about the upcoming surgery and trial. Everyone seemed to want to have memories of a normal holiday and not drag it down with thoughts of the future. We were OK with that as well. Debbie did mention to me once that she was feeling funny that nobody wanted to talk about what was coming, but she seemed to understand there was some denial (I mean, positive thinking) happening there too.

CHAPTER 16

January through February 2023 – Take Two

Debbie and I always wanted to stay at Red Lion Inn in Stockbridge, Massachusetts. It was a historic place and had some history for us as well. We had celebrated other anniversaries there, long ago when we had first moved to Winsted. It is a beautiful old inn with authentic New England cooking in the dining room and pub. I booked us a room for a night on the weekend before our forty-eighth wedding anniversary. We had a wonderful time there, wandering through the old hallways and spending some quality time in our special room. Debbie had put together a delicious charcuterie platter, and we cracked open a bottle of bubbly apple champagne, non-alcoholic of course.

We headed down to the dining room at our reserved time and found a quiet table near the back for us to celebrate our special time. We ordered some traditional fare and enjoyed dinner immensely. As we received our dessert, our server presented us with a greeting card envelope and said that dinner had been paid for by a friend. Tears were in our eyes as we read the card from our great friend Griff, who had driven up to the inn the day before with another friend and put his credit card on file to pay for the meal. What a totally thoughtful thing to do! That was perhaps the most special anniversary surprise we ever had, and we sniffled through the rest of dinner. That night we slept in peace and comfort in our big bed in the inn. We headed home very happy the next day.

On the 13th of January, we met again with Dr. B. and went over the arrangements for the infusion and surgery. We met with Dr. M., Debbie's surgeon, and her staff as well. Everything was looking positive and we were ready to go.

January 19th, Debbie had the first infusion of the test drug. It had to be administered in the infusion center connected to the Yale New Haven hospital. All infusions for the trial would be happening there too. There were three more Yale trips during January, including one standard MRI and one very special MRI. The second MRI was for a study that was being done to see if MRI could be utilized to see cancer cell metabolism. This was a separate study that was being done by the Yale University Medical

School, and they asked if Debbie would be willing to help with that. Of course, Debbie was willing to help, so she went through that test along with all the other poking and prodding that was being done to her.

During this time, Debbie was very watchful and aware of what was going on around and with her. She was worried a lot of the time, especially about the upcoming surgery. She tried to be tough, but I knew she had grave concerns. She was especially worried that something would happen and she would not be right after the surgery. She and I tried to dismiss that and be positive, but it kept bothering her.

February 1st, we checked into the hospital's hotel on the Yale New Haven campus. It was a special hotel for patients and family only. The room was nice and the staff very caring. We had the room for two nights so that I could stay there the night of surgery too. Brian took two days away from work and showed up at the hotel just a little after we had checked in. He would be at Yale through the surgery, and his calming influence helped us through many occasions.

The account of the next few days will be as clear as I can remember. A lot happened in this short time, and some of the facts and timing are a bit jumbled in my mind, so my story will be as close as I can get to the actual events.

The morning of the 2nd, we walked over to the hospital from the hotel. Literally arm in arm, we stepped into the main lobby and checked in. We were directed to the surgical pre-op waiting room and Debbie let them know she was there. Soon, the attendant came to get her, and we were led through many hallways up to the pre-op department. Debbie was quite nervous and not very talkative. Her normal lively sense of humor was put away for a bit. We were left for a few minutes to get her changed into a hospital gown. Brian, of course, waited outside the curtain of the "room" that was not really a room but a closet, covered by a surrounding curtain much like an emergency department that many people are familiar with.

Once dressed and in bed, we opened the curtains and waited. Dr. M. and her staff of anesthesiologists and nurses came in to see her and asked a few questions. Dr. M. told us what would happen during surgery. She told Brian and I that we could stay in the hospital and head to the neuro-ICU waiting room at some point later. It would be several hours, as the surgery was not a quick affair.

Shortly thereafter, I kissed Debbie as she was wheeled out of the little sanctuary. She smiled and gave me a thumbs up sign as she glided around the corner. Brian and I headed out to take a breath and find a place to sit with a cup of coffee. We expected a long day. We got one.

Much later in the day, and for the life of me I cannot remember the time, we were told that Debbie was nearly finished in surgery and the doctors were just finishing. We should remain in the waiting room and they would call us when we could go in to see her.

Finally, we were able to go to Debbie. She was in the neuro-ICU room and settled in. She was still asleep, but we could go and sit with her. Debbie was all hooked up to every sensor the hospital had, I think. She was breathing on her own and seemed small in the hospital bed. My eyes were quite misty as I had instant recall of the first time I had seen her after her first operation. The inflatable leggings were on her and there were tubes everywhere. I had to sit down after a quick bedside prayer of thanks that she had made it through OK.

Dr. M. came in shortly and spoke with Brian and I about the surgery. She told us that she had taken out everything she could, but that the tumor had grown into some very touchy areas. They had not been able to remove everything they wanted to, because the fibers were wrapped around some of the blood vessels near the motor center. Debbie had done well during the procedure, so Dr. M. was hopeful that she would be fine once she stabilized and swelling went down.

Brian and I sat and waited, nearly whispering to each other about what we had been told, hoping that Debbie would be all right. That news had not been what we wanted to hear. The nurses moved in and out of the room often, checking status on the machines and looking her over. The screens were showing good pulse and oxygen levels. Debbie seemed to be resting comfortably.

Debbie began to stir a bit later. As she woke up, we noticed a droopy look on the left side of her face. Her mouth sagged a bit and her cheek was also droopy. Her left eye was not open the same as her right. The nurses spoke with her and they tested her coordination, asking Debbie to raise her right arm and leg and then her left arm and leg. The right side was working fine, but the left side had no strength at that time. The nurses called it "weakness" of the left side. Debbie was sedated quite heavily, still from the surgery, but she was alarmed that her left side was not waking up.

Dr. M. came to the room and they checked again. She pulled us to the side and spoke to Brian and me about the situation. Dr. M. said that there appeared to be some weakness on the left side that she thought might be from swelling in the area where they had worked. She would be ordering a CT scan for overnight to determine if there was anything going on. She recommended that Brian and I go get some rest as there was nothing else we could do that night, and Debbie would want us in the morning. Debbie seemed comfortable and we decided that we could go in a little while.

Brian and I spent a short night in the hotel room. We tried to eat something and watch a bit of TV. I was feeling a bit numb and exhausted. Brian probably was, too, but he did not show it. I headed for bed and slept a fitful night until the light came in through the bedroom windows and I was awake. We headed for the hospital and after breakfast checked into the ICU waiting room. After a short wait, we were allowed to go into Debbie's room.

We greeted Debbie with a kiss and stood by the bed for a bit. She was awake now and her vital signs on the screens appeared to be normal. She told me she could not move her arm or leg and the doctors did not know why. Her face was the same as the previous night, and as she talked, her tongue got in the way of her teeth. Debbie's voice was weak and her words very slurred, so it was not easy to understand her, but her mind seemed to be pretty clear.

Dr. M. came in a bit later to see her. She checked the left and right motor skills again and spoke with Debbie about the weakness on the left side.

Dr. M. told Brian and I that the CT scan had been done. There was a tiny blood vessel that had been nicked during the procedure to get as much of the tumor as possible. Since the tumor was wrapped around the blood vessels that feed the brain in that area, she had attempted to get as much as she could without touching it, but one feeder vessel had been nicked. It was still bleeding a bit, and they were watching very closely to see that it did not get worse. This and the swelling in the brain from the surgery were causing some left side weakness.

Dr. M. explained that it was now dependent upon the swelling going down and the bleeding stopping on its own. They did not want to go back in to work on that vessel if they did not have to, as it would be hard on Debbie. We must wait and see. Dr. M. said she would be watching extremely closely and would make decisions as time showed what was happening. We thanked her and said we understood.

Debbie was in ICU for several days. This was partly due to a lack of beds in Dr. M.'s neuro-surgery department. Everyone told us this was lucky because the care that Debbie could receive in the ICU was much better than what could be done in a more standard room. Nurses continually checked on her and tested her motor skills.

During this time, Debbie's catheter was removed, and a new tool was used that we had not seen before. It was called a Purewick catheter. It was not internal but was set between Debbie's legs, and a tube ran out to a vacuum tank on the wall. I mention this now because it became vital to our ability to keep Debbie safely at home later.

As the days dragged by, Debbie's left side weakness did not improve. Though nurses and doctors poked and prodded and even cajoled Debbie into raising her hand and leg, or wiggling her fingers and toes, there was nothing really happening. They all told her, "good" when she tried, but it was not working.

We began to hear discussion about Debbie being moved over to the Grimes Center for rehab and further care. The Grimes Center is part of the Yale New Haven complex, but in a different building a few blocks away. This would be where Debbie could be given some therapy to get that left side working better and get her ready to go home.

Debbe remained in the ICU room, not being moved out to the other section. The decision was made that she would go directly from ICU to Grimes. Dr. M. came to me one day; by this time Brian had headed back to Boston, and I was there on my own with Debbie. Dr. M. told me that there were three possible scenarios that were at work here. The bleeding had stopped, or nearly stopped now, and the hope was that it was stopping on its own without further surgery.

Debbie's future depended upon these three things. The swelling could continue to go down, though it seemed that was done. The brain could compensate for the loss in that area and redirect signals to the arm and leg through another route, though at Debbie's age this brain elasticity may not have been possible. Or, given time, the weakness could be counteracted. Dr. M. was hopeful that these things could happen, but moving Debbie to the Grimes Center where therapy could be more intense was the best action to be taken. She said she would be over to visit Debbie often and continue checking on her.

There it was. Debbie had suffered what would be called a stroke during surgery. The brain bleed was the concern, and that is what had caused the weakness. Debbie's number one fear of the surgery had been real and had happened. This could determine her future.

The move to Grimes was not an easy one for Debbie. Her condition was very weak and moving her was very upsetting. She got a bit sick on the trip in the ambulance and was very embarrassed. It took a while to get her settled in her room and she was quite agitated. She was upset about the weakness and upset that she was not walking out of the hospital like everyone had promised. I understood completely and tried to calm the situation, but it was not easy.

Debbie was very alert by this time and very immobile. The good news was that at Grimes, I was able to stay with her all day and even all night if we wanted. We wanted. The first night, I could not stay as I had no supplies with me, and I felt I needed to get home for one night. We planned for me to stay after that.

The second day at Grimes Center, we noticed some swelling in the lower left leg when we were checking her out. The nurse noticed it, too, and called the attending physician. An ultrasound was immediately ordered for her. Upon checking with that test, it was determined that Debbie had a blood clot in the left leg, a very serious condition at this point. If it broke loose, it could travel to the lungs and cause an emergency. Within hours, it was determined that Debbie needed to go back to the hospital for treatment of that clot.

Another ambulance ride was called for and we headed to the emergency department for analysis and treatment. This ride went a bit better, though Debbie was still very immobile, and nobody wanted to cause issues with the clot. She was checked into emergency and into a first room for observation while a CT scan was scheduled.

The attendant wheeled her out into the main emergency department and through the halls of the hospital to the CT scan room. The scan was completed, and as they wheeled us back, it was determined that she would be moved to a different section of the department where they hold patients who were waiting for rooms. I was told I could stay and the staff gave me a cafeteria style chair that we squeezed into the tiny cubicle by the nurses' station. The space we were in was so small, I had to stand up and move whenever nurses would come to work with Debbie. But at least I could stay with her.

Debbie was given a heparin injection in the belly and then put on a heparin drip. Apparently, there was concern that the clot could be a problem, and they needed to get Debbie's blood thinned as quickly as possible. We were also told that we were just waiting for a room to become available for her on Dr. M.'s floor so she could be cared for more properly.

Thirty hours later, we were still in the emergency department cubicle. I spent the night in the cafeteria chair, trying to sleep sitting up while Debbie tried to rest in the bed. It was loud and active outside our curtain, so neither of us really slept. I felt so bad for Debbie during this time. She must have been quite terrified, but she did not show that much. As long as I was with her, she seemed to be able to handle most anything. She was a tough person, for sure.

Finally, we were moved up to Dr. M.'s floor and Debbie was in a double room. She was on a heparin IV at this point, and nurses were checking often to see that she was OK. There was no Purewick on this floor, so changing her was a bit of an ordeal. Debbie still had zero mobility in her left side and it was irritating her immensely. I was "happy" to see that she was getting a bit grouchy and asking for things. It was a good thing I was there, I think, so that I could mediate when necessary.

Brian visited and brought a nice dinner, but Debbie could eat little of it. She did taste a bit here and there but was not very hungry. Boy, she was grouchy, though.

Two days into that time and we were wondering what was happening. There was nothing for Debbie to do but feel glum and think about what she was up against. She wanted action and there was no action. We were told that she needed to stay in the hospital until they could get her off the heparin drip and onto a blood thinner, warfarin. She had to be stabilized on warfarin before she could go back to the Grimes Center. We began to worry that her room would have to be given up at Grimes and then we would not be able to go there. We were assured that Grimes would hold the room.

The next day, I got a call from Grimes saying that because Debbie was out of the room, they needed to move our things into storage until we moved back. They assured me they would have a room and hopefully a better one for Debbie. They already liked us and thought there was a room opening up that could house both of us if need be. The staff at Grimes was awesome and gave me a good feeling.

After five days back in the hospital bed, just waiting, we finally got word that Debbie would be moving back to

Grimes. The ambulance ride was easier this time, and we got to the center to discover that Debbie had been given a room at the very end of the floor, big enough for me to stay over when I wanted. It was quite comfortable and right next to a sunroom that we could use to get Debbie out of her room when we wanted. The staff was great and put up with Debbie's requests with mostly good spirits.

By this time, I was going home each night to Winsted and coming back each morning. Debbie's sister Tina determined it was time for her to come in from Pennsylvania and help however she could. She stayed in Winsted and helped at the house. Soon, she was traveling to New Haven too. We worked out a schedule for her to relieve me at Grimes and this was really helpful.

The Grimes Center was known for intense rehab to transition patients from the hospital environment to home. Debbie's case was one of trying to get her left side strengthened again and wake it up. Each day, the therapist would pick her up in the room and take her to the gym where they would get her standing and walking if possible.

I had many good conversations with the administrators at Grimes. During those, they explained that what had happened to Debbie was quite common with GBM patients, unfortunately. Grimes was where many of the patients ended up after surgery and often with some form of paralysis or disability. It was a difficult subject but very real in the perspective of the staff. Their role often became one of determining what they could work on with the patients to get them home or sometimes to another facility if the prospect of home life was too challenging. These discussions, I did not share with Debbie.

Debbie worked hard to get back up and going. She could stand up, once helped up. She learned to pivot. The therapist would use a belt to get her up and she would hold onto a ballet-style bar to stand. Some strength was coming back, and we hoped she would soon be up and around again.

The staff was told they must have two people to get her out of bed to go to the bathroom or get into her wheelchair. This was to be an issue with the center being quite short-staffed due to COVID. Within a couple of days, I was trained in how to get her up and given authority to get her out of bed myself. We did that quite a lot. Debbie became pretty good with pivoting quickly. She was driven to get back up and going.

Debbie's left arm was not responding very well to therapy. She could not get it to raise up or get the fingers moving. It was hurting a bit, so the therapists got her an arm brace to hold the wrist in a straighter position and keep the fingers open. This was more comfortable at least, though it did not help the immobility. Being left-handed made this even more of a burden. Debbie worked and worked to get some movement, but it was not happening yet.

We found out that the Grimes Center would be able to keep her there for just two weeks, and then she would need to head home. Their emphasis was on getting her up and standing. They determined that the arm was not going to get better soon, so standing would be most important. They even tried to get her to take a few steps along the parallel bars. She was so proud to stand at the bars and force her body to move forward a step or two. She was such a fighter; you could see the determination on her face.

The therapists trained me in how to get her up, how to pivot safely with her, and get her back down. I was not allowed to try to get her to walk, as this was deemed too unsafe at this time. We worked together in the gym and then again back in her room. Ultimately, I was able to help her get to the commode in the room and then back into bed. We were trained to move her to the right as much as possible, since her right side was unaffected by the weakness.

I thought it was very interesting, and at the same time a bit frustrating, that everyone called her left side weak. Why they could not say paralysis irked me, somehow. They never used the word paralysis, though I knew that was ultimately what it was. I guess they have guidance about that sort of thing and believe it might send a negative message to the patients. The reality was that at least for now, Debbie's whole left side was paralyzed and we did not know if it would get better. Debbie believed it would get back to normal with time and hard work.

The two weeks at Grimes were filled with days of therapy and then waiting for someone to help her. Debbie felt trapped there, I think. She wanted to be home where everything would be better. She wanted her body to be back to normal. She wanted to be able to get back to work and to relax in her house. She believed that she could beat the paralysis; it was just a matter of time.

Our time at the Grimes Center was coming to an end. The last few days, I stayed overnight with her in her room. I would get up in the morning with her and get her cleaned up. The staff taught me how to change her pants in bed, as the commode was not working out very well for her. She did not have the control to hold it until getting up and moving to the commode, so briefs had to be the answer. Later in the morning, Tina would come in, and I would head home for a few hours to do laundry and get things ready for Debbie to come home.

Brian came to visit the weekend before Debbie was scheduled to come home. We went through the house, and with the help of some great friends, we removed all the carpeting, moved furniture around or took it out, and we even opened up the doorway to the bathroom and hung a wider door. I measured all the doors we would need and determined they were wide enough for us to move through with a wheelchair. I put up some grab bars in the bedroom and dining room. We made the house ready for Debbie's access to the entire downstairs. Brian even built a temporary wooden ramp for the back door, and this worked for a few months until we replaced it with a permanent metal one.

On March 3rd, a month and a day after surgery, we took the ambulance ride from Grimes to home. We said farewell to the therapists and staff and packed up everything from

Debbie's room. Grimes had given us the tools we would need in order to survive safely at home.

Debbie was now able to get up with assistance and stand with a handhold. She could use the pivot disk to turn and then sit in a wheelchair. She was not able to use the commode, but I had been trained to change her. She required assistance to get dressed. Someone had to cut her food for her, but she could eat on her own using her right hand. It was life changing for sure, but we both knew we could manage at home, and I promised her we would make it.

The ambulance pulled up to our house in Winsted and Debbie was wheeled on the gurney into the dining room. We got her up and into a wheelchair. The attendants wished us luck and we thanked them for the safe ride home. They left and it was just Tina, Debbie, and me in the dining room. We were home.

CHAPTER 17

March – A Time of Change

Nearly as soon as the ambulance left, the challenges began. I got her into bed and we all took a breath. Debbie hated to be wet, so I changed her. She could not roll at all at that time, so changing her meant me pulling up her left side to slip the brief under her. At the Grimes Center, everyone called them briefs, I guess to make patients feel better about needing them. Debbie called them diapers, so I did too. She had no illusions about what they were. At that time, we chuckled a bit as I told Debbie that I had never changed pants on a girl before, at least alone. I was not even sure about the right way to clean her up.

It is difficult to explain how profound the difficulties we were facing were. Debbie was unable to roll or lift her buttocks up at all. She could not raise her left leg at all. Her left arm was rigidly tucked up toward her chest most of the time, but sometimes would stretch out. She could not move her hand, fingers, left foot, or toes. She could not sit up.

Debbie's right side was normal and already getting stronger to compensate for the weakness on the left. We had to use that strength to maneuver her in bed or in chairs. She could stand with nearly all her weight on the right foot. The left leg could hold some weight if it was positioned correctly. Debbie was able to pivot using the pivot disk, so that was how we would get her turned to go from bed to wheelchair, to chair, and back.

The one thing she had going for her was that Debbie truly believed she would walk again and use her arm and hand. She was determined to improve the use of them every day. She was a driven woman. Debbie had been one of the most independent people I ever knew before the surgery. She was able to use both left and right hands for much of the crafts and work that she did. She was always doing something with her hands. Now, she was challenged like never before, and the fight was in her.

The day after we came home, the VNA nurse arrived to determine what therapy and assistance we would need. They were comfortable with us immediately, and they were helpful with recommendations on how best to take care of Debbie's needs. They checked her vital signs and everything was looking good. A schedule was worked out that physical therapy and occupational therapy would happen two days per week, and a nurse would come at least once per week to check on her physical status.

On Sunday, two days after coming home, we held a welcome home party with family and a few friends. It was a little overwhelming for Debbie, but she showed everyone how she was progressing and that she could sit up and eat on her own. She moved from chair to chair to show how she could pivot. Her spirits were lifted high as family smothered her with hugs and love.

At one point, Debbie and I were in the bedroom changing her. We were trying to get her changed while standing as she gripped the grab bar I had installed by the bed. I turned for a moment to grab a wipe cloth, and in that second, she went down to the floor. Her left leg had collapsed under her and she lost her balance. Being on warfarin to thin her blood to prevent clots meant that any fall could be very dangerous. I was a bit stunned and I could not lift her on my own. We called for Brian to come and help. Debbie was mortified that Brian would see her with no pants on, but we had no choice but to use his help to get her up and into bed. Later we were scolded by the VNA nurse for not calling the ambulance. They told us that any fall was to be an immediate call for an ambulance because Debbie could have internal bleeding and we might not know it. This time we were very lucky. There was no issue other than a slight bruise on her hip where she fell.

At this time of our home life, Debbie did not want anyone else changing her. That was tough because at Grimes there had always been options for others to change her when she needed it, though they often made her wait until they had time to do it. Once we were home, she did not want to wait. I think we changed her eight times a day some days. It was grueling work for both of us.

Debbie's wake-up routine went the same every day. First, I would warm some water for a sponge bath. I would bring that in and then wash her legs and feet. She often worked on raising her left leg and bending it as she got stronger. Then I would change her. She chose which pants she wanted to wear and we put those on before sitting her up. Then we sat her up and washed her upper body. She chose her shirt and we put that on.

Then, we sat on the bed side by side and I asked her if she wanted to hold hands. This was a ritual we did where I put her left arm over my arm with her hand cupped over mine. Then I would raise my arm and move it around, stretching further as we warmed up. We would bend the arm and straighten it, then loop it around and go up and down. Every time, at the finish, I moved her hand up so she would brush her nose, like she was giving the old Italian gesture of "screw you." This nearly always made her smile and I would act like it hurt me. It was a special moment in the day that we shared, and the touching was good for both of us.

Debbie was a very particular person. She had always wanted things the way she wanted them, and that's it. Generally, this did not always affect me, but now I was her arms and hands, so I was doing what she was used to doing. This approach applied to many parts of her day, but perhaps none more than the nighttime ritual that began to take shape, and much to my distress took hold. Each night, we wheeled into the bedroom and changed with her standing up at the grab bar we used for the commode during the day. We changed her into pajamas every night. It was interesting that many of her rituals involved certain movements and exercise. I could never argue that too much because I felt it kept her muscles in better tone.

Once the pj's were on, we put on her night brace for the left arm and we wheeled to the bed facing the corner. This way, Debbie could get up and move to the right. We were always moving to the right, her strong side. She would carefully sit down on the bed and we would swing her legs up and into bed. Then, a pillow must go under the knees and one under the feet. Cover her up. Next, a pillow for the side, tucked just under her butt, but not too far up. A smaller particular pillow goes next under the left arm to hold it just so. Another pillow would go under the head. Our bed was a fancy Sleep Number job with raisable head and feet. The feet had to be raised to just the right height and then the head just a bit. "No, lower please." Always please and thank you, bless her. Then find her little friend, a stuffed furry thing we called "Scrunjee." The sheet and top blanket would be put on. Then, her favorite survivor's blanket to keep things cozy. The doorbell button used to summon me was hung on the side rail just by her pillow. The bed table needed to be wheeled into place with tissues, lip balm, water, and her cell phone. (She checked the time throughout the night.) Finally, I had to give her the lip balm to wet her lips for the night. A quick check of everything and we were done. We ended with a sweet kiss. Thank goodness, always a sweet kiss. This ritual was done every night as long as she was in our bedroom. She did not appreciate it when I listed the steps, so I only did that when I was mad.

Once, we got all the way through and she said she was wet again. Everything came off and we started over. Good grief! This was when we installed the Purewick, purchased direct from the company and a true lifesaver (at least a true marriage saver).

On Monday the VNA physical therapist came for her first visit. We spent that first hour trying different things to see what Debbie could do. They needed to form a baseline of where we were starting. The therapist was happy to see that Debbie had some capability for standing and pivoting. It was decided that we would focus on that for the first few visits. Debbie worked so hard during those visits. She was typically exhausted and ready for a nap when the therapist left. There was no giving up in Debbie. She pushed herself and the therapist every time they met.

One driving factor for Debbie was the bathroom. We spent a great deal of time talking about and doing bathroom activities. It was too difficult for Debbie to get to a commode for "number one," but she hated, really hated, "number two" in a diaper. She forced herself to use a commode for that. Whenever she had the slightest urge to go, she would say, "I need to take a walk to the bedroom, Tim." Which was code for using the commode, which we had put in the bedroom because there was a very handy grab bar in place to make the transfer from wheelchair to commode. She had only two accidents in all the months she was home. But in order to avoid them, we had many false alarms. She would sheepishly say she couldn't go, after we had rushed into the bedroom and made the change. She talked about going to the bathroom more than anyone I ever knew. But I really could not blame her, and it was not a terrible thing for her to get up and work her muscles every now and then. For a long time, Debbie would allow only me to change her or accompany her to the commode. This was a challenge, but I accepted it. Ultimately, her sisters forced the issue, but only several months into the new way of living.

Later in the week, Debbie's occupational therapist met with us for the first time, and Debbie was very happy that someone was finally working with her arm and hand. Sandy, the therapist, not the sister, massaged her arm, and they found that Debbie's left shoulder was dropping a bit. That was what had been causing her pain during the day when she was sitting. We found a sling on Amazon that would help and I ordered it immediately. Debbie and Sandy worked on the hand as well. They massaged the fingers and tried to get them to straighten out and become a bit more flexible. It was hard work, and Debbie was in pain some of the time during these sessions. Sandy was great and figured out ways for them to get the arm and shoulder working together more. Debbie was certain she would gain the use of that arm and hand again and never gave up.

On Sunday, March 12th, Debbie and I shoveled her into the car, and we headed to the Yale hotel for the night. The next day there was an MRI and an appointment with Dr. B. to discuss the medical trial. Debbie had been working so hard to get her mobility back that we had not thought too much about the trial but were very anxious to find out what was going to happen. I had been trying to temper the idea a bit, as I was not sure Debbie could really handle the stress of going to Yale every week for infusions, moving from car, to wheelchair, to infusion couch, and back.

The MRI was very challenging due to her lack of mobility. The nurses and I had to stand her up and pivot her onto the MRI bed and lying still was not easy. Debbie made it through, though, and we headed up to Dr. B.'s office.

Dr. B. was not able to see us that day. His associate, Patrick, met us instead. It was not in the normal examination room. Patrick said that the MRI was indicating that much of the tumor had been removed and the site was clear. He tested Debbie's mobility and talked with us about how it was going at home.

Patrick talked about the clinical trial requirements for a few minutes. He explained that there was a sliding scale regarding patient self-sufficiency and mobility. He carefully explained to us that due to the weakness on the left side and resulting lack of mobility, Debbie was too far down the scale to allow her to continue the trial. Debbie was devastated. I had felt that the trial would be too much for her, but I had been reluctant to tell her. In this case, I was glad it was the medical staff telling her and not me. She was angry at Patrick, and no matter how I framed the situation, she was mad and disappointed.

Patrick told us that the option for treatments was typically to move to Avastin, an infusion that could be administered in the Torrington Yale treatment center. Avastin was the standard treatment at the time for recurring GBM, so it was natural to start that protocol as soon as possible.

Patrick explained that we would work with the staff at Torrington for the treatments and continue to come to Yale New Haven every two months for an MRI and appointment with Dr. B. We left that appointment drained and disappointed, both knowing for sure that the trial drug would not be possible for Debbie. Our ride home was very quiet.

Physical and occupational therapy continued at home over the next few weeks. Each time they visited, the therapists gave me ideas for improvements around the house or for Debbie's comfort, and I ordered and installed more bars and a sliding shower chair. The therapists were a bit amazed at the quick actions in many cases, so they gave even more ideas. They were great with Debbie. Debbie continued to work hard to improve her strength.

Avastin treatments were administered every two weeks. We would drive to Torrington, and I would sit with her as she had the blood work and infusion. The staff was great and played into Debbie's positive attitude greatly. They talked about getting her better and stronger. I bit my tongue sometimes when I felt they were too positive, but Debbie ate it up. I know now that was her right, and it kept her going.

The staff at Smilo in Torrington was exceptional. People don't become cancer infusion nurses by accident. These people were among the most positive people I have ever met. One nurse, Abby, was immediately Debbie's favorite, and she was bubbly and caring. She was also an expert at her job and was the one everyone called when the IV needle insertion was a problem. We called her "Stabby Abby." She was gentle and kind. All the other nurses were special people too. I cannot say enough about how they treated Debbie, making sure she was happier when she left than when she came into the center.

On March 24th we headed back to Yale to have her stitches removed and the wound examined. Dr. M. met with us and we talked about the Avastin treatments and how she was doing. Debbie was still upset about not being in the trial, but Dr. M. calmed her a bit, explaining the challenges she would have faced. The wound was healed and Debbie was happy to know that at least.

March 30th was Debbie's sixty-sixth birthday. We celebrated at the house with the grandkids making her a cake.

I played it up by holding a fire extinguisher near the cake because there were so many candles. Debbie's crooked smile was broad that night, and everyone was delighted to celebrate with her.

Around her birthday, while everyone was visiting, Liz and Megan arranged for Debbie to receive a manicure and pedicure at home from a traveling nail specialist. This was a very nice thing for them to do and made Debbie feel great. She was the center of attention for something fun, and that was also great. We had another one for her a month or two later before we were able to get out for one ourselves.

Debbie's crooked smile was a very important part of her recovery and longevity during these tough times. Her sense of humor actually got sharper and sharper as time passed. She would say some very funny things and the timing was right. It was a delight to have her smile and laugh with therapists, nurses, family, and friends. To this day, I don't know where that came from; somewhere down deep, I think. It must have been some survival mechanism at work inside Debbie. We often joked as she was being changed or dressed in the morning or moved from chair to chair. She always tried to keep it light. In some ways during this time, there was almost a childlike personality that came through. Debbie was very loving and lovable. I was always amazed that she never really showed anger.

Throughout the next several months, Debbie's sisters Sandy, Tina, and Lesa all came to visit for extended periods of time. They were invaluable to us in so many ways it is impossible to say how much it meant to us. Each of them had special skills and talents that were put to use throughout each day. They cooked, cleaned, did laundry, helped move Debbie around, listened to whatever Debbie and I were saying, gave advice, and lived with us. It was astounding to both of us how much each of them gave up of their time and energy. Debbie was grateful, and I will be forever thankful for their presence in our lives.

CHAPTER 18

April through June –
Making the Best of It All

On April 2nd Debbie and I joined Colleen on a trip to Greenwich, CT, to see Peter Noone. It was quite a trek, as Debbie could still barely get into the car, let alone attend a concert. But I wanted to do everything in my power to give her meaningful experiences. We arrived in Greenwich and found a parking spot right in front of the theater. There was a dinner scheduled with other "Noonatics" just down the street, and we manage to get her wheelchair down the crooked old sidewalks and into the restaurant. Debbie was beaming as we gathered with old friends. The dinner was great, though Debbie had some trouble eating. We cut up her burger and she was just fine.

Back up at the theater, there was a challenge getting her down to a spot near the stage. We moved some chairs around, and she ended up nearly under the spot where Peter would be performing. That crooked smile was broad and teeth were showing as the warmup tunes began. I had to move back to a seat near the back in order for there to be room for her and Colleen, so I kept watch as best I could to make sure Debbie was not in trouble during the show. She loved it! Peter checked her out a couple of times and she felt special. When the show was over, we made our way back out to the car, and Colleen came running after us saying that Peter wanted to see her. That made Debbie's night. We spun back around and headed in to see him. He spoke to Debbie for a few minutes and told her that he was happy she could come.

Therapy continued at home. Sandy came up with some creative ways to get Debbie's hand moving. One day, she taped all her fingers to Debbie's fingers and moved them around, picking up some training cups that Debbie had on the table and just getting those fingers moving. Another time, she worked with Debbie on an exercise where Debbie would lean forward toward the table, Sandy would put a cup in front of her hand, and Debbie was to pull back to move that cup off the table. It was quite hilarious when Debbie realized she could cheat a little bit and move her whole body back to do it. She laughed and smiled at us when the cup dropped off the table. Nobody let on that we knew she cheated, but we all laughed about it.

About this time, we noticed that Debbie often asked for her yellow writing tablet. She struggled a lot at first, as she tried to write right-handed. She wrote pages of notes about things she thought of. Debbie's mind was always at work. Thinking about work or pottery or grandkids or what we needed to buy at the store or what needed to be done for the ambulance. I could read her writing, though I am not too sure others could or even she.

She wrote a list of who needed thank you notes for the nice things people had done. I don't think she missed anyone. One day she asked for her laptop to be set up for writing thank you notes. I helped her set up a template that she could use to write the notes, and sister Sandy helped retrieve them from the printer. We would write out the envelopes and Debbie would stuff them. She sent notes to everyone she could think of and we heard later people really appreciated them.

Sometimes Debbie would get quiet and she would be just staring and thinking. We asked her what she was thinking and she would say "nothing." We never knew all that Debbie had on her mind, but I am certain it was a lot. She would get tired just thinking.

Naps were every day and usually quite long. For a couple of hours in the afternoon, she would sleep peacefully in the darkened bedroom. I think, and she said, that the naps were usually better than her sleep at night. Only heaven knows what she thought about during the night, but it was a lot.

Jen, her physical therapist, was working with Debbie on standing and walking. We got a special walker for her called a hemi-walker. It was made for people who could only use one hand. It was a bit like a cane with four spread feet. It was solid enough to bear Debbie's weight along with her right foot. Jen strapped on a leg brace to help stabilize Debbie's left knee, which was her weakest point. They put on a web belt around Debbie's waist that Jen could hold onto. Then, Debbie would stand up out of her wheelchair and walk with the aid of Jen. The first time they did it, Debbie walked a couple of steps and then felt unsteady, nearly falling, but Jen caught her. That scared us all, so from that point on, whenever Debbie walked, we had someone walk right behind her with a wheelchair for emergency purposes. Debbie never fell again. She did great and we took some videos of these exciting moments. It was funny because Debbie would ask, "Are you getting this?" and would be focused more on us getting the video than her walking. She was so proud and we were proud of her.

Debbie was pivoting so well by this time that we no longer used the pivot disk. Debbie and I had a routine of how we would move from one chair to another, or from the bed to the chair. She got stronger and stronger, and her right side really compensated for the left side's weakness.

Debbie eventually got more used to transferring from the wheelchair to the front seat of the car. This allowed us to make a few short trips to things she wanted to see. We visited RRDD1 a couple of times, and she tearfully spoke with coworkers about what was going on, promising to be back at work as soon as she could. We visited Nutmeg Pottery, and she went in to see what was going on. It was too early for her to start working in clay, but you could see her eyes sparkle with new ideas popping into her head.

Avastin treatments continued and Debbie felt more positive that she was going to get better. Her drive to improve was constant. We got into a daily routine too. In the morning I woke up around 6:00 a.m. and did my exercises, showered, had some coffee, and read a little bit. I went in to get Debbie out of bed at around 8:00 or 8:30. She used to ask to get up earlier, but I could not get up and get her right up or I would have been behind for the rest of the day. I had to always be at least one step ahead of her throughout the day just to make sure she had what she needed when she needed it.

As she got stronger, Debbie set a goal for herself to dance at our niece Sarah's wedding which was coming up on Memorial Day weekend. It was a lofty goal for someone in her current condition, but it drove her to work hard. Debbie always set goals and worked toward them. I think it was something that kept her going.

I was always trying to think of things that would make her happier, or bring some meaning, while trying to stay reasonable. There were things she wanted to do that I did not see how we could do, but I tried to find ways to compromise or adjust those wishes. I started thinking about the one thing that might make her happiest. She had been talking about going on an Alaska cruise for years. It was top on her list of things she had been wanting to do before the cancer hit her. I thought about it and wondered if I could still make it happen if we went soon enough. Finally, one night I asked her if there was a way to do it, would she want to go. She answered me, "You mean like a final wish?" That hurt both of us and I said no, just would she want to go. She did not really say anything more about it and I dropped it. I felt a bit heartbroken that Debbie had answered in that way, but she was just being honest with me.

I did come up with a way we might travel, though. I hooked up a computer to our large screen TV and we could get YouTube on it. I found a YouTube video series on a man from Miami who traveled all over the US in his camper, with his wife. It so happened that about the time I found his videos, he was preparing to set out on a life-long dream trip to Alaska. We began to watch these videos and looked forward to each new video to catch up on where they had been. It was great and Debbie loved it. We watched it together and talked about what they were seeing and doing and how beautiful it was.

Other times, we watched Hallmark together. She loved the emotion and warmth of the stories, even though we got to the point where we knew what would happen next in nearly every movie. It did not matter to us. We just sat together and enjoyed the shared moments.

In May I decided to get a tattoo. This was something I had thought about for years and I felt strongly that it was time. I had an idea for the artwork. It came from a special gift a friend from the Elks had given me recently. She gave me a coin that had a passage from the Bible: Philippians 4:13, "I can do all things through him who gives me strength." I loved this passage, and I believed this was what was giving the strength to do what I had to do with Debbie. I worked with the tattoo artist to design a cross and a yellow rose (the special flower of Debbie and me) all arranged with a ribbon flowing through them. It was a beautiful design, and I had it tattooed on my right arm where I would see it every day. Debbie was not sure about it at first, I think because she had not known me to be very religious in recent years. I found that I was becoming more and more spiritual and religious, even becoming a true believer again. I knew this was what I wanted, and Debbie was OK with it once she saw it. It meant and still means a great deal to me.

Treatments, therapy, naps, and trips to doctors took up much of our time for the next few weeks, right up until Memorial Day. I found a beautiful pants suit for Debbie to wear to the wedding. She loved it too. It was white cotton pants with an expandable waist and comfortable coral-colored jacket. An orange blouse topped it off. And it looked great with the sneakers Debbie always wore. I bought a matching coral-colored shirt and tie for me. By this time, I was down to one-hundred-sixty pounds, so I also needed new pants. We were matched in our outfits.

We traveled to Pennsylvania and stayed at the same hotel as everyone else. We made the room work. Hotels were not really set up to handle Debbie's disability, but I took whatever we needed, and with a bit of adjustment here and there Debbie was able to handle it. When we were at hotels or hospitals or out to eat, if we needed to use the toilet, it was quite an ordeal. We just did what we had to do, though. It was one of those things.

The day of the wedding was spectacular. The wedding was outside, and the reception was in a beautifully renovated barn. There were over a hundred people there. Most of the family made it in, and many of Sarah's and Donnie's friends. The ceremony went well. Debbie and I found our table and settled in. Everyone was enjoying it. We had brought with us a special platter that Debbie had made for Sarah and Donnie. It had their names stamped on it and was glazed in beautiful wedding colors. She had finished it just before she had gone for surgery, so was waiting a long time to give it to them.

As the dance music began to play, I looked at Debbie and she at me. I slowly and carefully wheeled her through the crowd of tables up to the dance floor. Her sister Sandy stood behind her holding the wheelchair, and I slipped into place and helped her stand. For a whole slow song, we held each other, and she danced at her niece's wedding. Debbie's sisters were around, not too close, but all watching. Sandy was trying not to start bawling, but Debbie and I were both teary-eyed. She had reached her goal. We danced.

June was a month of routine. Avastin treatments came and went. One big change after the Memorial Day trip was that the VNA determined they had done everything they could to help Debbie at home. She was upset, but they told us we could still get therapy; it would just have to be at a therapy center. We could hardly argue that since we now were getting into and out of the car more easily. We bid farewell to the staff of VNA who had helped so much. All of them were great and very motivating to Debbie. We promised to keep in touch, and they told us they would be around if we ever needed them in the future. As was often the case, Debbie presented each of these special people with a pottery piece she had made. Often these were her angel impressions or a little dish to remember her by.

Debbie started therapy at the Winsted Physical Therapy Center in town early in June. We met a great therapist, Paige, who took over her walking practice right away and had some new ideas that helped strengthen her right side, while continuing to stabilize her left. They practiced standing and walking, with me always a step behind, wheeling the chair along just in case she needed it. She did not need it. Debbie was proud to be walking more and counted the steps each time, proclaiming the new number each session. Once again, Debbie's keen sense of humor showed through on many occasions. She would sometimes try to trick Paige or take a short cut that, of course, Paige would catch and make her do over. It was funny to watch the interaction between them.

They worked on her arm, too, though it was not coming along as well as the leg. Debbie never gave up trying to get that arm and hand to cooperate. It was a major frustration to her that it would not listen to her, no matter how she talked to it. She did not let it get her too down though. She just kept trying.

During the previous couple of months, Debbie's partners at Nutmeg Pottery determined that moving the studio from its location on Main Street in Winsted to a new space in the Old Hurley Industrial building in New Hartford would save the studio nearly $1000 per month in energy cost, and the rent would remain just about the same. At first, Debbie felt like the studio was abandoning her and she fought the idea. She worried that the change might be bad for the studio and for her. But as she thought more about it and her best friend at the Studio, Pam, told her more about it, Debbie realized it would be for the best.

Debbie was determined to have her things moved to the new studio, too, and everyone agreed. She supervised the packing of her tools and partially finished pieces. I packed them in boxes and trucked them down to the new location, just eight miles away. I helped move quite a lot of the shared equipment and supplies too.

One day late in the move, I took Debbie to the new space and we moved her boxes in. As I unloaded them from the truck onto a hand cart, I had some very strange feelings. The Hurley building is where I had worked for twenty years when I was working for the Ovation Guitar company and we were based there. As I pushed the carts up the hallway to the elevator that would take us to the second-floor workspace, I realized I had pushed hundreds of carts up that same hall and even to that same space when I was working as a guitar maker. I wheeled the boxes into the studio where Debbie was waiting, and we talked about how odd it was to be back there. Debbie felt it, too, as she had worked upstairs for a year in the Hurley Spring company. It was somehow fitting that we had come back around to this place.

Debbie liked the new space immediately. Pam and the other women had made sure she had a spot that was easily accessible for her wheelchair, and she could work if she wanted to, whenever she had the strength and time to do it.

Debbie wanted to make pottery again. With only one hand and always seated, this would be quite a challenge. I learned once more that you cannot tell Debbie, "No." She just fights harder. One day there I had the wrong attitude and was paying more attention to something I was doing on my phone than to what she was trying to do. I told myself that if she wanted to make pottery, fine, she could go ahead and do it. If it did not work, well then Debbie would just have to realize that and find something else to do. At the moment, I did not realize, no, honestly, I did not care, that this hurt her deeply. She did not say anything to me right then. But later that night, she scolded me for being so cold. I realized then that I had been very wrong to do what I had done. With misty eyes of realization, I promised her that we are still a team and that any time we were at the studio in the future, my attention would be on her, and I would be her hands and legs if she needed me. We hugged tightly that night.

One area of concern for Debbie had always been her personal appearance. She always had beautiful clothes and liked to dress up. She was an avid collector of broaches and necklaces and always wore a broach that fit the subject of interest for the occasion. She also cared a great deal for her hair and nails. Once we were a bit more mobile with the car, we occasionally went to the nail salon she always used in Winsted. It was a big deal to get her into the shop from the car and then into the chair for a pedicure. We did this together and she felt much better for doing it. Her nails were beautiful, and she often received compliments from therapists, nurses, caregivers, friends, and family about how nice they looked. We even had a chance to get to her favorite hair salon when Jonathan cut her hair and I took photos. These experiences were challenging but very beneficial to her self-image. We managed to get to the nail salon a few times before the end of the year.

Later that month, I had a colonoscopy that had been put off for some time due to Debbie's scheduling and personal needs. I did not want to cancel it again; well, I wanted to but I knew I shouldn't. Tina and Sandy were in town, so I was able to do the preparation routine the night before, and Tina took me to the procedure. Sandy stayed with Debbie while Tina was with me. The doctors removed several polyps and one larger one that required leaving a clip inside. They told me I would need to come back in four months again for another colonoscopy to check it out. That was that.

As we were getting around a bit more, I wished we could visit Boston to be with the family there from time to time. It was not possible for us to visit Brian's house because of the stairs. It was not possible to visit my father or brother for the same reasons, though they lived only a short distance from Boston. For a couple of years, we had been talking with Brian about the possibility of having a place of our own. Originally, it was to be a stand-alone house built new in their back yard in Dorchester. But COVID and red tape had put that off too long. The cost of building had sky-rocketed, too, since COVID. Brian approached me one evening back in the spring about us taking over the bottom-floor apartment in their three-apartment house, located just through the backyard of their own house. He told me it would be vacant after the school year, and he felt it would be a nice fit for our needs. I loved the idea!

I had discussed this plan with Debbie a few times and she was very cool to the idea. She did not understand why I would want to move away from our house. I attempted to explain that it would be just another place for us to go, so we could get up to Boston for visits. She was very suspicious that I was not being totally honest about my intentions. She thought I was trying to trick her into agreeing to move. In all honesty, I was thinking about me in this scenario, because I believed I would not want to stay in our house in Winsted when Debbie was gone. I could not tell her that, though it was somewhat obvious.

After several discussions explaining the benefits of the second home, Debbie relented, though always suspicious of the true reason for it. We went ahead with plans to set up the apartment once it was unoccupied. I truly believed that Debbie would enjoy being able to go up there for visits too. I knew it would be good for both of us. Then, later, it would be good for me.

CHAPTER 19

July and August –
An Active Time

As the summer progressed, we hired a caregiver from a local service to come in once per week to watch Debbie while I went to my friend's house for Wednesday night dinner with the boys. CC was a great help and quickly fell in love with Debbie. She was watchful and careful with Debbie and they became great friends. She kept busy all the time, washing, sweeping, and even doing laundry. She was a friend to Debbie and Debbie looked forward to seeing her. She continued working with us through the end, and I am very thankful for her.

July was more of the same. Avastin treatments were going well. Friends were visiting now, and it was nice to be out on the back porch for the summer. Debbie loved to sit out there and look at her garden. We fed birds in a feeder hanging off the barn. Debbie called the birds "little piggies" because they would swarm the bird feeder and eat all the seeds so quickly. It was very entertaining.

Debbie's goal for working at RRDD1 was to make it to July 1st, the beginning of the new fiscal year for that organization. It meant that she would collect a pension for the previous year and that was a huge item on her mind. Though she had not been physically able to work there since February, the board of directors was able to keep her on the books using her sick time built up from previous years. The staff of RRDD1 acted nobly to keep things going on their own, and the members of the board were on hand to help when needed. This was a testament to Debbie's commitment to them and theirs to her. I was amazed that everyone stepped up to the plate and made it work. Finally, Debbie realized that it was time for her to step down officially, and I helped her write a letter informing the board of her retirement as administrator. This was harder for Debbie than anything she had done so far. She still did not want to leave work; it still meant so much to her. With tears, she put the letter in an envelope that I then delivered to the office. This was on July 15th.

We spent a couple of days at the new pottery studio where Debbie started some new pieces. The first was a large bowl. It was one of her "floppy" style bowls that started as a slab and was formed within a very large bowl. She took parts of the clay and folded them in and out so that the top had a floppy appearance when completed. Then the bowl sat inside the large bowl to dry into the final shape. Her friend Pam made the large slab, and Debbie and I laid it into the bowl mold. Then Debbie formed the folds to her liking. We took a picture of her holding this piece in her lap, a huge, crooked smile on her face. This was posted on social media and received many likes and comments from friends who were astounded that she was back making pots.

July 28th we headed back for an MRI at Yale. During this one, the nurses said I could stay in the room with Debbie during it. So, I was able to help get her onto the MRI bed and then sit in a chair right near her. The machine was deafening, so we could not communicate during it, but she knew I was there. Debbie liked me to be with her all the time at this point. I liked being with her too.

In the appointment, Dr. B. told us that, once again, "there was no change," and we left for home in a happy place. The Avastin was working, and Dr. B. said it seemed like it might actually be shrinking the remnant of the tumor, which was rare but not unknown. Debbie was thrilled to hear it. She started thinking about beating it again.

Aaron arrived one weekend in early August and we put up a new metal ramp for the back door. Debbie, especially, had become concerned that once bad weather hit Winsted the wooden ramp would no longer be safe. I'm sure she was right. A new ramp was found at a friend of a friend's house and it was donated to us. What a special gift. Aaron and I pulled the ramp apart and designed a new layout for it. We put it up at the back door and it worked fabulously for the remainder of the time we needed it.

During August, Debbie continued working with the therapists, we had to switch because her favorite, Paige, had to go back to teaching. Paige's husband and partner in therapy, Dave, took over and continued the walking practice religiously. By this time, Debbie was walking in the hallway because the gym was not large enough. She would walk up the hallway two or three times, with me following of course. Then Dave would take her into the "torture chamber," Debbie's name for his therapy room that hand a bench where he would stretch her left leg and work her left arm. These sessions were the highlight of Debbie's week, and she wished she could go every day. Dave always walked us out to the car after the session and helped get her into the front seat and load the chair. He was a very caring partner in Debbie's good health.

Debbie continued to work at the studio when she had energy. We worked together as a team on some small platters and leaf dishes. We pressed out some more angels and other small goods, especially for use as gifts to people that helped her. These times were much better there than they had been. Our teamwork produced some nice pieces.

In early August the apartment became available. Brian, Liz, the kids, and even her father who lived right around the corner ripped through the place. They cleaned it all up and painted every surface. Brian sent us a video tour of the new space, and both Debbie and I got excited about it, me more than she.

I found a ramp for the Boston apartment on social media, and Brian picked it up and installed it before our first time to the apartment. It worked out great and made Debbie feel at home on our very first visit.

When we got there, the house was all furnished with beautiful hand-me-down furniture and a brand-new motorized recliner. Debbie loved the recliner and settled right in. The apartment was fresh and clean and the colors were just right. The first night, Brian and Liz brought down dinner from their house, just through the backyard and up the hill. It was magical to be able to stay there and just relax.

We had a study that, originally, I thought would be for me but thought better of it and told Debbie it was to be our shared study. I set up a table for her to work on her crafts or laptop by the windows, overlooking a beautiful tree and the street. I set up a ham radio workstation in a closet in that room so we could work in there together.

There was plenty of room to move around in the apartment and the doors were all wide. The bathroom was a little bit challenging, but we made it work. It is remarkable how adding a wheelchair to the mix makes things more complicated. What seems so simple becomes a project to be solved. We did it, though, and Debbie was a real trooper. She knew I was very happy there.

The bedroom was set up with a massive king-size bed. This one did not have the feature of raising head or feet, but I was confident we could make it work. If we could manage the rest of the standard wake-up and nighttime rituals, Debbie felt good enough about it. I just had to use some more pillows than we did at home. Once in bed, she slept well. We had a second doorbell call button for Boston, so she was able to alert me when she needed me in the mornings or after naps.

Back at home in Winsted, Debbie was commissioned by our good friend Meagan to make a platter for her son's wedding in October. We started this platter, much like the one she made for Sarah and Donnie, earlier this year. That was a new goal, to finish the platter in time for the wedding.

CHAPTER 20

September and October – Summer Is Over

One weekend in September, all the Kessler siblings were able to visit our home at the same time. We got a great photo of Tina, Lesa, Eddie, Sandy, and Debbie out on our back porch. It was a memorable occasion to have them all together. Terri, the only missing sister, was missed much by the others and her memory was toasted. This family has been through a lot in the last few years, and to have a moment together to remember the good times was important. We were very glad it happened.

On September 21st, Debbie and I headed for the Boston apartment again. This time, to celebrate the fiftieth anniversary of our first date. I wanted it to be something special. Aaron even flew in from Virginia to be with us for it. I bought Debbie fifty yellow roses and had them put all in one vase. It was eye-popping and just what I wanted to give Debbie. She loved it, and we had a great weekend.

During that trip, we worked on the platter for Meagan's son's wedding. Debbie began stamping the words and names she wanted into it. Along the way, I noticed that several of her letters were backwards and she was having a difficult time seeing it. After some rework and creative adjustment, we got them all fixed up. I was a bit alarmed by the trouble, but I kept it to myself and we laughed about it.

We also began noticing that Debbie's naps were getting longer in the afternoons. Sometimes, they lasted three or four hours. And her appetite was decreasing. These signs were not significant at the time, but we noticed them.

Back home, on September 30th, we attended the Fall Foliage Festival in Winsted. A few months back, the VNA therapists had arranged for us to get a motorized wheelchair for Debbie, thinking it would give her more mobility and we would not have to push her everywhere. That had not worked out as planned because Debbie's left eye depth perception was, unbeknownst to us, not very good, and she could not drive the chair around the house without bumping into things. The one and only time we ever used that chair was to drive down the street to the Foliage Festival. It was quite hilarious to see Debbie try to drive it along the curb in the road as I stayed by the side to turn it back to the right direction along the way.

Once we got down to the fair, I let her drive a couple of times. The first time she had the controls alone she drove right into a booth and almost knocked the table over. Too much for her to handle, I guess. So, I took the controls and walked alongside her. That worked fine.

I noticed that she was having a difficult time recognizing people she had known for years as we bumped into them along Main Street. I guess we could chalk it up to overstimulation, but it concerned me a little bit. We eventually said all our hellos to friends and made our way back up the street. Debbie was happy to have gone, but it exhausted her and she took another long nap.

That was the last time she used the motorized chair. I hid it in the back room and she never asked about it again. I called the chair company and they picked it up a couple of weeks later.

In early October we asked Debbie's friend Pam to finish glazing the wedding platter. Debbie had tried to paint the letters, but her dexterity with the right hand was not what it needed to be. Pam did a wonderful job, and we presented the finished product to Meagan one day at the house. She loved it, especially knowing what she knew it took Debbie to do it. That was the last commissioned piece Debbie made, a gift for a friend.

After Debbie's first Avastin infusion in October, as we got into the car, Debbie told me to head for Joann Fabric store in Torrington. I asked why and she just said, "I need some things." I drove to the store and got her out of the car and into the wheelchair. We had not been in this store for many months, so I was not sure what she had in mind.

She pointed to the fabric section and we wheeled up and down the aisles. Debbie was looking for something in particular. I asked what we were looking for and she pointed at the baby blanket fabric. I asked, "What is this for?"

Debbie said, "Sarah's baby."

"Debbie, I don't think we can do this right now."

Debbie got quite angry at me. "I'm tired of you telling me I cannot do things. Stop telling me no!"

I was taken aback by this. I wheeled her around, silently. She was mad. I was mad. I bit my tongue hard. Debbie found the fabric she wanted and we picked up the roll of fabric. Then we headed for the backing and then the filler. She found what she wanted, and we headed for the cutting table where a young clerk cut the fabric to the specifications Debbie told her. She put the pieces in a pile, and we headed for the checkout counter and paid. I tried not to say anything more. Debbie had a determined look on her face that told me we were not discussing this.

When we got home after the shopping trip, I got her ready for her nap and we settled in. The bag of baby blanket supplies sat by her recliner. We spoke no more of this for some time.

Finally, a few days later, I took the bag upstairs and put it with many other things we had bought and not used. I figured there was no way it would ever be used, but it had been something Debbie had in her mind that she could somehow do, one-handed, or not.

On October 14th, RRDD1 threw a retirement party for Debbie. It was held in the office of the facility. Many of her friends from work attended. Our friend Griff catered the event, making fresh pizza in an oven outside. Aaron's and Brian's families were there and Debbie's sister Sandy. It was a great affair in which Debbie received a plaque from the board and a citation from the state, presented by our great friend Representative Jay Case. There were congratulatory cards from many vendors and gifts from the staff. The party was a great success. Debbie was the center of attention, taking to the floor in her wheelchair to tell little stories of many occasions that had happened. She was funny and happy.

Later in the month, after her second infusion of the month, Debbie was scheduled for an MRI. We made the standard trip to New Haven expecting the usual. After the MRI was completed, we headed up to see Dr. B. in his office. He knocked on the door as always and came in to make pleasant conversation.

He checked Debbie's coordination and asked how it had been going recently. "Have you noticed any changes?" I mentioned that there were a few little things that seemed different lately. As we swung around to the computer, he said, "Let's take a look at the slides."

On the screen was the August slide next to the slide for that day. He explained and pointed, "There appears to be a change in this area." We could see some shadowing, wispy shading in the area of the tumor. There were traces, or rays, moving out slightly toward the outside and rear of the cavity. There was some more shading toward the center of the picture than before.

Dr. B. stated, "It appears the Avastin is no longer holding back the tumor. It is becoming resistant." Both Debbie and I looked at the two slides with a combination of disbelief and dread. Dr. B. went on to say that this is a change for the negative. He turned back around to face Debbie and said that we have the option of stopping treatment or going on with the Avastin. There is no chance for another clinical trial that would be helpful.

"What would you like to do?"

Debbie choked a bit on her breath, trying to compose herself. She said, "What's the choice?" Dr. B. repeated the question.

Debbie said rather flatly, "Avastin"

Dr. B. seemed not to understand, so I interjected, "Debbie wants to continue the Avastin."

Dr. B. said that it might be helpful to continue it. It would not be curative, but it would be helpful to reduce swelling, and without it, the tumor would likely advance more quickly. He stated that he could support this because it would be helpful to continue, for now. He said he would order four more infusions, and we would schedule another MRI for December and discuss options.

Our worst fears had been realized, was all Debbie and I could think as we left the hospital that day and headed back home. Debbie sniffled in the car on the way home. I could think of little to say that would ease the shock as the new situation set in. We had not expected this, but we had. We did not think it would come to this, but we knew it would. Our minds reran the conversation over and over into that night.

I put Debbie to bed that night and I think she cried. There was nothing I could think of to do to fix this one. I felt out of options and pain set in.

Sandy and Lesa were visiting during the month, on and off. During a conversation between Debbie and Sandy in the living room, the trip to Joann Fabric came up. They talked about how we had bought the fabric and it had been a bad scene.

Sandy and Lesa went upstairs to check things out and found the bag with the fabric. Sandy remembers Lesa bringing the bag downstairs and saying, "I think we can work on this together. Sandy can sew, and I can do some of the stitching."

Debbie had a new goal. The sisters would finish this baby blanket in time for Sarah's baby shower, scheduled for the Saturday after Thanksgiving. Could it be done? With determination and Debbie's leadership, they believed it could. The three sisters started work on it that week.

We brought Debbie's sewing machine, a very advanced embroidery machine, downstairs and put it on the dining table. Sandy read the manual and practiced sewing a few things to get used to it. The fabric was brought out and cut to the right size. I ran back to the fabric store to pick up safety pins that would be used to hold the fabric in place while it was sewed.

When I got back with the pins, Debbie walked the girls through the process of pinning the top, filler, and back together to form the blanket. Sandy and Lesa sewed stitching around the edge of the blanket to hold everything together permanently. We took photos and video of the work the three did together. They showed a combination of determination and joy on the faces of the three coworkers. It was truly a special time that I had not believed would ever be accomplished. Silly me.

By the time Lesa left to go back home, the blanket was ready to have the outside trim hand-sewed in place and the darts sewed to hold the interior of the blanket so it would not bunch up.

Sandy took the blanket back to her house with her and promised to work on the outside trim. Lesa asked to have the chance to sew the darts later, so she could have more to do. The project was well in hand, and it would be done by the time of the baby shower. That was a promise from all three.

CHAPTER 21

November and December – What Is Next?

The next week, sister Sandy arrived again and would spend a while with us. Debbie went back to Smilo Torrington and received another Avastin infusion. The nurses were exceptionally positive and talked about her being back again. That was a good thing. We met with Dr. C., Debbie's oncologist at the Torrington clinic. He knew some of what had happened, and he knew the results of the MRI. He seemed to have another opinion of the outlook. He recommended that we see a friend of his at Dana-Farber, the world-renowned cancer center in Boston, to discuss the case. He said he would make the referral to his friend and would contact Dr. B. to let him know. I felt awkward, like we were going behind Dr. B.'s back, but I also figured that if there was any hope for Debbie, we had to try it. We would make contact with Dana-Farber and see what comes of it.

Two days later, with Sandy joining us, we went to the Cohen Brain Tumor Conference that we had attended the year before. I had tried to hide this from Debbie a few weeks before, but she knew it was coming up and forced the issue. She really wanted to go.

We arrived at the hotel in Hartford for the conference and signed in. This time Debbie was in a wheelchair and was obviously the most advanced case in the room. Everyone was thrilled to see her again, and we met several people who had been there the last time.

The main address was given by one of the leaders in brain cancer research from Sloan Kettering institute. His talk was about the successes and failures of recent cancer clinical trials and the state of brain cancer treatments. The timing of this topic was a bit shocking. Sandy, Debbie, and I listened intently about the three main types of brain cancer and treatment of each. The worst, being GBM, has had little improvement over the past twenty years. Specific mention was made of the failure of Avastin to produce the results that had been hoped for and expected. There were other trials going on, including one using immunotherapy (likely the trial Debbie had been scheduled to be part of). There was some other information, but it was lost on me at that point.

After his talk I looked at Sandy and then asked Debbie what she had thought of the presentation. "Very promising," was the answer.

"Very promising?" I asked as I looked back at Sandy whose eyebrows were raised in disbelief. "Yes, I thought it was good for the future."

What a sweet, dear person to answer in that way. I dared not go into what my thoughts were on it. We quickly changed the subject as people were getting up to grab the lunch that was being served. We continued to meet and great other folks, and more nurses and caregivers gravitated toward Debbie.

After lunch, there was a breakout session for patients and caregivers held in two different rooms. Sandy elected to stay with Debbie in the patients' session, while I headed to the caregivers' session. We talked about our experiences and our patients, how strong they are, and what they are going through. Some spoke about what we were going through. I spoke about the stage we are at and the importance of positive thinking/denial, two sides of the same coin I believe.

We left with a positive feeling and a lot of well-wishes. I was glad it was done. I know Debbie was happy to have gone.

Debbie was back at physical therapy the next week, working as hard as ever to improve her walking and stretch her arm. She never gave up on therapy and prayed it would never stop.

On Wednesday the 15th, we headed up to our apartment in Boston. Thursday morning was our appointment at Dana-Farber. Because of her advanced stage, the center had gotten us right in. I had sent releases to get her case materials up to them before our visit, so they were ready for our appointment when we got there. Brian took the day off from work and went with us to this appointment. I felt it would be good to have a second set of ears and eyes at this point.

We ended up meeting with two doctors, associates of the friend that Dr. C. had recommended. They discussed Debbie's case and her options. They told us that Dr. B. has a great reputation in the field and is well-known even in Dana-Farber. They explained that there may be an option to start chemotherapy again, but they would contact Dr. B. and defer to him on that point. Basically, we got nothing definitive or new from them. The good news, if there was anything good, was that they concurred with Dr. B. and thought he was doing the best for her in her condition.

We headed back home with solemn hearts. Nothing would come of what Dr. C. had thought might be a breakthrough. In some ways, I felt we had been led down a fruitless path. I also respected Dr. C. for at least attempting to help. And we did end up with a second concurring opinion, which was at least some comfort that no stone had been left unturned.

Thanksgiving was no comfort this year. Debbie and I planned to go to Boston to be with Brian and Liz for the weekend, but Debbie was not feeling well enough to travel. She was weaker and was sleeping a lot. On Thanksgiving Day, we sat at home. Debbie cried most of the day. She was feeling really miserable. I contacted some friends at our Elks Lodge. They always made dinner for a local homeless shelter and some shut ins. They were thrilled to be able to bring dinner to Debbie and me. They showed up at our door with two turkey dinners with all the fixings and even an apple pie made by our friend, the one who had sent the coin with the inscription that inspired my tattoo. The two friends that brought the dinner came in and talked with Debbie a while and made her feel a little better.

Saturday after Thanksgiving was the date of Sarah's baby shower. The blanket had been done for a few weeks, and Sandy had it at her house to be wrapped and presented to Sarah. The three sisters had completed it together, and it was a beautiful blanket. It would be a gift that Sarah and her baby would cherish forever.

On Friday, after Thanksgiving, Debbie said, "I want to go to Sarah's shower." I was surprised. She had not been feeling well for days and was quite weak. Could we make it happen? With luck and determination, I thought we could. I decided to take Debbie on Saturday morning and bring her home that night. Staying overnight anywhere at this point was very challenging, much more challenging than just getting her into the car and to the event.

The shower was being held at the VFW where Sarah and her husband Donnie volunteer and socialize with good friends. This was in Scranton, about two hundred miles from our home. Early Saturday morning, I loaded the car with any supplies we might need throughout the day, but no overnight supplies. We got Debbie into the car and settled her back in the passenger seat for the long ride. She was quite sleepy and so slept the whole ride to the shower.

We arrived at the VFW hall early. Sandy and Lesa were there to help us get Debbie out of the car and into her wheelchair. We wheeled her into the building and into the bathroom to get her changed for the party. Sandy guarded the door so nobody would be surprised by a man in the lady's room. Debbie was so happy to be there and be wearing a pretty outfit and jewelry. It was a happy moment when I wheeled her back out into the event hall, which was decorated beautifully for the shower.

We found a spot at the end of one of the long tables where we could put Debbie's chair, and I left her to be with friends and family for a while. She was beaming. She had made it to the shower, once again beating the negative thinking that should have prevented such an accomplishment. Another goal met.

I stayed out in the lounge area while the party went on so Debbie could enjoy it without me hovering over her. The party went on for a couple of hours. Finally, the gifts were presented to Sarah. The last gift was presented to her by Debbie, Sandy, and Lesa—the blanket that had been so lovingly made by the three sisters. Sarah was amazed and shocked by the present. It was a beautiful blanket made much more beautiful by understanding how it was done. Lesa even gave her photos from the dining room sessions. The moment was spectacular. How could I still have doubted that Debbie would accomplish what she set out to do?

After the party and another trip to the bathroom to get changed for the trip, we shoveled a very exhausted Debbie back into the car for the ride home. The trip back to Connecticut was easy and uneventful. Debbie slept most of the way, and we got her into bed for a peaceful night of rest.

After Thanksgiving, Debbie had some issues with her eyes that seemed to affect her ability to cry. She told many people she could not cry anymore since Thanksgiving. She wanted me to make an eye appointment for her to see about getting new glasses. She was having trouble seeing too. She kept asking, but I knew there was nothing anyone was going to be able to do about her eyes. My belief was the tumor was beginning to press on her optic nerve and perhaps the back of the eye. I could not fix it.

The first week in December, Debbie's physical therapy did not go as well as it had been. She was weaker and unable to finish the three times up the hall before going to the torture chamber. Once on the bench, she suddenly got nauseated and threw up her breakfast, barely getting a waste bin under her chin to avoid making a mess. She was very embarrassed, and Dave gently worked her left shoulder to calm her down. They did not do the rest of the leg stretches.

On Wednesday the 6th, Debbie had another Avastin infusion as Smilo Torrington. We explained to Dr. C. what we had found out at Dana-Farber, and he said it was good that we went. Her infusion went on normally and the nurses were kind.

That night Debbie attended our annual radio club dinner that I host at the end of each year at a local restaurant. Debbie was funny and happy to be there and everyone enjoyed seeing her. It was nice to have the friends get to see her and we wished all happy holidays.

During the month, CC began to talk to Debbie about making pies and cookies. She had never made a pie and asked Debbie if she would help her. It was a joy for Debbie to be in the kitchen with CC, and they made several pies together.

Later in the month, Debbie and Sandy made meatballs. What a funny picture it was to see Debbie in an apron squishing the hamburger into balls and putting them on the tray. She loved cooking, and Sandy had given her a great gift.

Debbie's next infusion on the 19th was the last that Dr. B. had scheduled. We took some of Debbie's small pottery pieces with us and gave them to the attending nurses, thanking them for the wonderful work they had done with Debbie. They were quite taken aback to receive such a personal gift from Debbie, and we left with high emotions.

Typically, we had always been able to schedule the MRI and doctor appointment at Yale the same day. It was a lot for us to make two trips to Yale on separate days, and they were always able to accommodate us. This time, however, we were scheduled for an MRI on Saturday, December 23rd and then to come back on Tuesday, December 26th. That is rotten scheduling in anyone's book. But that was it. I tried to make it better by telling Debbie we would head up to our Boston apartment right from the MRI on Saturday. Then we would spend Christmas there with Brian and family. We would head back to Yale on Tuesday morning right from Boston.

Debbie was very tired now. She slept long hours in naps. Physical therapy on the Thursday before Christmas was hard. She did not have much energy for it. We gave Dave a piece of pottery for him and Paige, thanking them for all they had done. We hoped to see him after Christmas.

Saturday arrived and we got Debbie in the car, with lots of gifts and supplies for Boston too. We headed down to an empty Yale campus. It was nearly abandoned, for the holidays. The MRI went normally, with me helping to get Debbie on the bed and sitting with her. Debbie did a fine job of being very still, so the test went quickly.

We were off to Boston right after getting dressed. It took an extra hour or so to get there, but we made it without any issues. Brian and the kids met us at the apartment. They had gone out that day and bought a Christmas tree. It was decorated with many ornaments from the past that were not on our other tree at home, still up after two years. Debbie eyes sparkled, though I was not sure how much of it she could really make out. She was complaining a lot about how her eyes were bothering her now.

She sat in her favorite recliner, and the kids sat nearby, enjoying the company and the Christmas spirit. I put the presents we had brought with us under the tree and the place looked festive.

Christmas Eve was very nice. Liz made a big dinner and brought it all down to our apartment where we all ate together. There was an underlying sadness that could hardly be detected, but I think everyone felt it. Debbie ate a bit and napped a lot.

Christmas morning, we had brunch at our apartment. Very tasty and filling, it was just right. We all opened the presents under the tree, and Debbie sat in her recliner taking it all in. She was not very talkative, but it was obvious she was happy to be there. The party moved from our house up to Bob's house (Liz's father) and we stayed behind to relax. Debbie had a long nap.

Tuesday morning came early for us. We needed to be on the road by 8:00 in order to make the appointment, and we had to pack up first. We got on the road and retraced our steps to Yale New Haven from Boston. Again, the campus was very sparse, so parking was very easy. We made our way up to Dr. B.'s office and waited to be called in.

Dr. B. knocked lightly and came into the examination room. He asked how things had been lately and we told him some of the things we had been experiencing. He did not bother checking Debbie's mobility this time. He had a visible agenda. He seemed a bit resigned this time, rather than the positive nature he normally showed.

Dr. B. turned to the computer and said, "Let's look at the slides."

The October slide and the slide from the 23rd were up, side by side. He pointed out how the tumor had continued to advance, more aggressively now. There were brighter areas of solid color in the tumor cavity, with a more solid area toward the center of the picture. The areas that were rays before were now solid tracers. There was some bright red in sections where there had been nothing.

He turned back to us saying, "The Avastin is no longer effective. The tumor is growing aggressively." Sigh, "I cannot recommend continuing the treatments at this point."

"What does that mean?" Debbie asked.

"Well, our option is to do nothing, or to get therapeutic care." Dr. B. said.

"You mean hospice?" I asked.

"Yes, I'm recommending that you contact our hospice coordinator. My nurse will be here in a moment with some details for you and we will take care of it."

"Will they tell us what to do? We have worked with Litchfield VNA. Can we use them?" I asked.

"Yes, we have worked with them and they are very good. Debbie, Tim, I'm sorry to tell this to you. It has been wonderful working with you both, and I wish you all the best. You can call anytime if you have questions."

With that, Dr. B. shook our hands and bowed. He was always so positive in the past. It was hurting him deeply to be having this conversation, I could tell.

"Thank you, Dr. B. You have been great to work with, and we appreciate all you have done for Debbie. Thank you."

Dr. B. left and his nurse came in immediately to go over the details with us. They would be writing an order for the VNA to take over with hospice. We had to sign paperwork to get that rolling and the nurse had that all ready. Within a few minutes, all that needed to be done there to close out three years of work was done. I felt empty.

We both cried as we headed home this time. This would be the last trip to Yale. No more MRI. No more appointments at Yale. No more infusions. No more trips to Smilo Torrington. Home we went, to stay.

By Thursday the 28th, Litchfield VNA Hospice had been contacted by Yale, and they were on the case in a very effective and efficient way. They reached out to me by phone and scheduled an appointment to visit us and go through a questionnaire to get things going.

CHAPTER 22

January through February 2024 – Hospice

To Debbie, hospice meant only one thing. For months she had not said the word or talk about the possibility. Dying was not discussed, except in a passing moment, usually with her sisters. Her entire being had been programmed to live. She had even kept going to physical therapy with hopes of improvement long after most would have known things were not getting better. Debbie was a powerful force.

Now, with hospice in the house, I think she embraced it. At the very first meeting, Debbie had asked the question about getting a bed. When it came up, I was so surprised that I told the nurse who was going through the questionnaire to hold on for a day or two while we discussed it.

Later, I asked where she wanted to put the bed and she said, "Right here in the living room," pointing to where she was sitting in her power recliner (we had one for Winsted too). I told her we would have to take down the Christmas tree that had been up since that first November weekend three years ago. She said OK, just like that. That was it. The tree was taken down and we put it away lovingly. It had done its job.

In its place I moved the plant table from the dining room into the living room and put up a Christmas light line in the window in the shape of a triangle, to remind Debbie of the tree that had occupied that space for three years. The plants made the living room really alive too.

One thing I noticed about hospice is that they get things done, like right now. The next day after asking for the bed, it was delivered and set up in the living room. This was the 3rd of January. Debbie's sister Lesa had ordered a special comforter for it and Tina ordered matching sheets. It looked very cozy, not like a hospital bed. But it had all the adjustments we would need for caring for Debbie from either side as time went on.

Hospice also sent over a "comfort pack" the very first day of care. It contained several prescriptions for pain and comfort that would be ready whenever it was needed. I did not even know what was in it until the nurse went over it with me a few days later.

I did not fully understand why Debbie wanted the bed, but I think it was to protect me from having her in the bedroom as time went on. In the later days of us being in the bedroom, I had been sleeping in a cot at the base of the bed. I could not sleep in our bed with the head and foot raised as high as Debbie needed it, but I knew it meant a lot to have me close by. I put up the cot every night and took it down every morning.

Once Debbie moved into the bed in the living room, I slept on the couch right near her. By this time, Tina and Sandy were both staying with us, and soon after, Lesa came in to stay. They all stayed and went as they needed when they had to deal with something on the home front. But my memory is that they were all there nearly all the time. What dedication!

Debbie was surprised when people stopped poking and prodding her. She had a few bad dreams about people coming to take blood, and we assured her that would not happen again. She asked when the next infusion would be and we said no more infusions. Debbie's state of consciousness began to shift once all the medicines were dropped. One by one, we stopped the blood thinners, the thyroid medicine, the anti-seizure medication, and the sleeping pills.

Dreams and daytime reality mixed sometimes. Debbie's sense of humor remained, amazingly. Her sisters would take turns with me sitting with her and just talking or listening to the TV. I think her eyesight had failed dramatically by then, but she did not say, would not say. Hallucinations came and went too. Some of her funniest comments came during and after these episodes.

January 10th was our forty-ninth wedding anniversary. I did not make a big deal about it. We mentioned it, but Debbie was not taken by it. I think the fiftieth anniversary of the first date meant more. We let it go by without fanfare.

This stage of Debbie's life was not the most important in the scheme of things. She never gave up, though, not even then. She fought to keep awake and aware of her sisters and me. Each day she slipped a little bit more, losing strength.

By now, Debbie's sisters had taken me off changing duties and took care of her themselves. It was a relief to me, but it felt very strange not having to be there for that every few hours. They changed her pajamas with the help of the hospice caregiver. They fed her dinners when she would eat. They kept water for her on her table for when she would drink.

CC continued to come every week, and she sat with Debbie while she was here. I could not take that away from either of them. CC had become one of the family, another sister if you will.

On about January 30th, Debbie stopped eating. When she did eat, she was not keeping it down, and that bothered her more than being hungry. She was in bed all the time at this point, and she just seemed to lose interest in it.

On February 1st drinking stopped too. She was not swallowing well by that time and drinking was too difficult. We fed her water from a syringe when she asked for it, which was seldom.

Debbie liked to have her sisters or me sit with her and talk about good things in the past. She was beginning to see other people in the room too. At first, just shadows, I think. Then she seemed to be able to pick out relatives that were gone. At night sometimes I would hear her having a conversation with someone. I could only hear her side, answering someone or talking with them. I just listened, knowing it was not for me.

I wondered how long this could go on. Debbie was not in any pain or discomfort. She needed nothing from the care pack. She was just fading.

On Saturday, February 3rd, Debbie was beginning to be agitated more. We asked about using the care pack and were given instructions on how to do it. That night, she began having breathing problems. At about 8:00 p.m. she began a series of deep breaths, followed by stopping altogether for many seconds. I stayed up all night with her holding her hand as this continued into the night. I spoke with her about how well she had done and how we were all here for her, but she could not answer. She squeezed my hand and kept on going. By 2:00 a.m., I was exhausted and could not stay sitting anymore. Sandy was sleeping in the recliner in the other room, and I asked if she could sit with Debbie for an hour. I lay down on the couch and closed my eyes. I prayed for resolution and peace for Debbie.

I got back up, and by about 6:00 a.m. the breathing changed. At 10:00 we called hospice and asked for a nurse to stop in to see Debbie. Shortly thereafter a nurse who was new to us came and examined Debbie. She reported to us that the end was coming and Debbie was doing OK. She explained that more medication could keep her comfortable and that it would be all right to give more if she needed it.

After she left, I contacted Aaron and Brian to let them know what was going on. They assured me they would be available if I needed them and they were OK too.

I texted Debbie's best friend, Colleen, who had been coming a lot to see Debbie. I suggested she should come as soon as she could. She did, arriving at about 1:30. She sat with Debbie for a while and she spoke to her and prayed. I know Debbie knew she was there. She finally left at about 2:40, saying she thought it was time for her to go.

Lesa and I moved to the back sitting room and we were listening to some music and talking. Sandy was in the kitchen. Tina was sitting with Debbie. At 2:55 Sandy came tearing back into the back room and told us Tina said she thinks Debbie was gone.

We all rushed around the bed. As I ran in, I saw the most serene, peaceful expression on Debbie's face. All lines were gone. All fear and tension were released. Debbie had won the battle. My beautiful girl was gone.

I was so proud of her. She won her last battle and let go when she was ready. What a powerful person she was for doing that.

We called hospice, and the same wonderful nurse came back to our house to take care of Debbie's last needs.

The battle was done, over three years after the first shot was fired. She was my outlier. I thank God for Debbie and for all of those who helped us through this greatest challenge of her life.

Epilogue

As I finish this story on the back porch of our house in Winsted, I feel Debbie's presence all around me. I know she is looking out for me, and her love continues for me as my love continues for her. She was an amazing person, bigger than life. Her inner strength was something to be experienced.

During the three years of our journey through glioblastoma multi-form, I often struggled with the difference between positive thinking and denial. I have determined that in the case of brain cancer, there is no struggle, no difference. It does not matter what you call it. The patient has every right to use whatever mental tools are necessary to keep going.

Debbie's positive thinking was what kept her going through all the worst times she experienced.

What was most important was love. We shared fifty years of our lives and I only wish we had fifty more. It felt like we were just getting started. But I also know that those fifty years were so special that I must be very thankful for them and the memories they created.

My hope for the reader is that you may find some small tidbits of information or an idea that might be helpful in your situation.

We were told by doctors and other care professionals that we should not try to calculate our chances or our future by the statistics. We are each our own statistic, and we must live our own life as long as we can.

I miss Debbie every day and I am thankful for the time we had. These last three years were the fullest and most intense times of our lives.

I think we made the most of the time we had.

I thank God for the help we had from Debbie's family and our boys and their families. We could not have made it without their love and assistance through it all.

About the Author

Author Tim Angell lives in Winsted, a small town in Northwest Connecticut. He is a retired corporate financial reporting manager, but has had many interests over the years, including amateur radio, woodworking, cycling, golfing and writing. He is inspired by everything around him and tends to dig deep into whatever subject catches his interest.

Love of family has always been the primary interest and his wife Debbie was his most vocal inspiration. Tim has two boys, their wives and six grandchildren to continue pushing him to keep going.

Tim's civic background is in Boy Scouting as a leader, the Benevolent and Protective Order of Elks as a lodge and state officer, and Amateur Radio club president.

This is his first book, though there are ideas for others kicking around in his mind.